contents

introduction

This ... has been ... by a... experienced paramedic instructor to guide you through your first aid course, and to provide you with a reference for future years.

Most people will find the information in this book useful and informative, but it cannot replace 'hands on' training in the vital skills of dealing with an emergency situation.

Effective emergency treatment before professional help arrives can go a long way to reducing the effects of illness and injury, and indeed save someone's life.

Taking part in a first aid course and using this manual may be the most important decision you make in your life...

Edition 5.01

IMPORTANT
This manual is designed as a learning guide to a full first aid course, it cannot replace 'hands on' training in the vital skills of dealing with an emergency situation.

If you suspect illness or injury, you should always seek professional medical advice.

DISCLAIMER
Whilst every effort has been made to ensure the accuracy of the information contained within this manual, the author does not accept any liability for any inaccuracies or for any subsequent mistreatment of any person, however caused.

first aid

the aims of first aid

Preserve Life

Not only the casualty's life, but your own as well. Far too often only one person's life is in danger when the emergency services are called, but by the time they arrive there are more. If you put your life in danger, you can end up fighting for your OWN life instead of the casualty's.

Prevent the situation from Worsening

The skilled first aider must take action to prevent the whole situation from becoming worse *(e.g. removing dangers such as traffic or fumes),* as well as acting to prevent the casualty's condition from deteriorating.

Promote Recovery

The actions of a first aider should, after preventing things from getting worse, help the casualty to recover from their illness or injury.

priorities of treatment

All animal life needs a constant supply of oxygen to survive. If that oxygen is taken away for any reason, brain cells will start to die within 3 to 4 minutes.

The priorities of treatment are therefore aimed firstly at getting oxygen into the blood stream, ensuring that the blood is circulating around the body, and then preventing the loss of that blood. If this aim is achieved, then the majority of casualties will still be alive when the ambulance arrives.

The first priority with any patient is to make sure the **Airway** is open and then to check they are **Breathing** normally *(A and B).* If the patient is breathing normally, this means that their heart must also be beating, so blood is being circulated around the body. As the **A** and **B** check is carried out first, we call it the *'primary survey'.*

Once you are happy that the casualty is **Breathing** normally and oxygen is being circulated around the body, the next priority is to deal with any major **Bleeding**, because you need to maintain enough blood to circulate the oxygen around. After these steps, the next priority is to deal with any broken **Bones (BBB).** The check for bleeding and then broken bones is called the *'secondary survey'.*

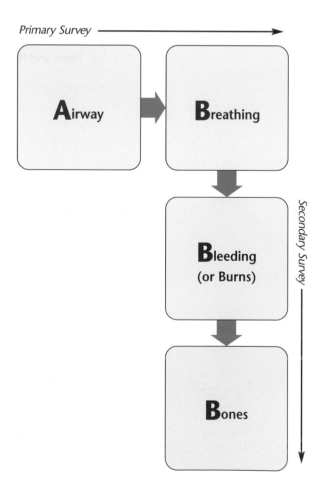

Primary Survey ⟶

Airway ➡ **B**reathing

Bleeding (or Burns)

Bones

Secondary Survey

multiple casualties

*The **BBB** rule can be used for multiple casualties, to decide who needs treatment first. A rough 'rule of thumb' is that the casualty who is the quietest needs treatment first, where as the one making the most noise (trying to get your attention) is the least serious!*

It is important to have an action plan for emergencies. This flow chart guides you through the actions to be taken when dealing with a patient. All the topics, such as the recovery position and resuscitation are covered later in the book.

DANGER?
Look for any further danger.

 NO

YES

Remove Danger
Make the scene safe. Do not take risks.

Response?
Shout and gently shake or tap the casualty.

 NO

YES

History
Find out what has happened.

Signs and Symptoms
How does the patient feel or look? Try to work out what's wrong.

Treatment
Remember – if you're not sure, always seek professional medical advice.

Help!
Shout for help but don't leave the casualty yet.

Airway
Open the airway by tilting the head back and lifting the chin.

Normal Breathing?
Look, listen and feel for no more than 10 seconds.

If you're not sure if breathing is normal, treat it as though it is **not**.

YES

Secondary Survey
Check for bleeding, injuries and clues *(see page 10)*.

Recovery Position
- Recovery position *(see page 11)*.
- **Dial 999 if not already done.**
- Monitor Airway and Breathing.
- Keep the casualty warm.

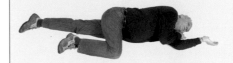

 NO

Dial 999 Now
(If not already done)

Resuscitation

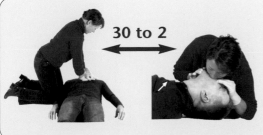

30 to 2

- Give 30 chest compressions, then 2 rescue breaths.
- Continue giving cycles of 30 compressions to 2 rescue breaths.
- Only stop to recheck the patient if they start breathing **normally** – otherwise do not interrupt resuscitation.
- If there is more than one rescuer, change over every 2 minutes to prevent fatigue.

resuscitation

the chain of survival

In order to maintain the oxygen supply to the body a person must be breathing, and their heart must be 'pumping'. If either of these two functions stop, the brain and other vital organs will quickly deteriorate, and brain cells will start to die within 3 to 4 minutes. Unless urgent action is taken to circulate oxygen around the body, this will inevitably result in death.

The most common cause of cardiac arrest in adults is 'ventricular fibrillation'. In these circumstances the best chance of restarting the heart is by using a 'defibrillator', which is carried on all emergency ambulances in the UK. For this reason, an emphasis is placed on summoning help and dialling 999 as soon as possible. Of course, the heart and brain must be kept oxygenated until the defibrillator arrives; so early Cardio Pulmonary Resuscitation (CPR) is vital if a casualty is to recover. These actions form the 'links' in the chain of survival (see diagram).

Early CPR
CPR is performed to keep the vital organs alive until help arrives.

Early Advanced Care
Advanced life support treatment is given to stabilise the casualty's condition.

Early Access
Help is summoned so an ambulance (with defibrillator) can arrive as soon as possible.

Early Defibrillation
A controlled electric shock is given to try and restart the heart.

Cardio Pulmonary Resuscitation (CPR) – primary survey:

D Danger – *make sure it's safe and find out what's happened*

- Check that it is safe for you to help the casualty. Do not put yourself at risk in any way.
- If possible remove any danger from the casualty, or if not, can you safely move the casualty from the danger?
- Find out what's happened – and make sure you are still safe.
- Check how many casualties there are. Can you cope?

R Response – *are they conscious?*

- Gently shake the shoulders and ask loudly 'Are you alright?'
- If there is no response, shout for help immediately, but do not leave the casualty yet.

A Airway – *open the airway*

- Carefully open the airway by using 'head tilt' and 'chin lift':
  - Place your hand on the forehead and gently tilt the head back.
  - With your fingertips under the point of the casualty's chin, lift the chin to open the airway (see diagram).

B Breathing – *check for normal breathing*

Keeping the airway open, check to see if the breathing is normal. Take no more than 10 seconds to do this:

- Look at the chest and abdomen for movement.
- Listen for the sounds of breathing (more than the occasional gasp).
- Feel for air on your cheek or movement of the chest or abdomen.

If the casualty **is** breathing **normally**, carry out a secondary survey and place them in the recovery position (pages 11 and 12).

Airway blocked by the tongue.

Airway cleared by tilting the head and lifting the chin.

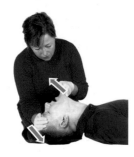

Gently shake the shoulders and shout.

Gently tip the head back and lift the chin to open the airway.

*NOTE: In the first few minutes after cardiac arrest, a casualty may be barely breathing, or taking infrequent, noisy gasps. Do not confuse this with normal breathing. If you have any doubt, act as if it is **not** normal.*

if the casualty is not breathing normally:

Ask someone to **dial 999 for an ambulance** or, if you are on your own, do this yourself; you may need to leave the casualty. Start chest compressions as follows:

- Place the heel of one hand in the centre of the casualty's chest, then place the heel of your other hand on top and interlock your fingers *(see diagram)*.

- Position yourself vertically above the casualty's chest with your arms straight.

- Press down on the breastbone 4 to 5cm *(1½ to 2 inches)* then release the pressure without losing contact between your hands and the chest *(chest compression)*. Ensure that pressure is not applied over the casualty's ribs. Don't apply pressure over the upper abdomen or the bottom end of the breastbone.

- Compression and release should take an equal amount of time.

- Do 30 chest compressions at a rate of 100 per minute.

- Now combine chest compressions with rescue breaths *(below)*.

NOTE: Ideally the casualty needs to be on a firm flat surface to perform chest compressions (not a bed). One way to remove someone from a low bed is to unhook the bed sheets and use them to slide the casualty carefully to the floor. Get help if you can and be very careful not to injure yourself or the casualty. Do not move the casualty if you do not think it's safe to do so – remove the pillows and attempt CPR on the bed instead.

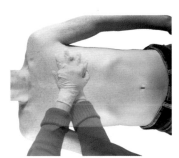

Look, listen and feel for normal breathing.

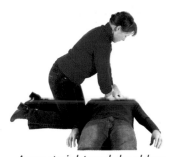

Place the heel of one hand in the centre of the chest, then the other hand on top.

combine chest compression with rescue breaths:

- Open the airway again, using head tilt and chin lift.

- Nip the soft part of the casualty's nose closed. Allow the mouth to open, but maintain chin lift.

- Take a normal breath and seal your lips around the casualty's mouth.

- Blow steadily into the casualty's mouth, whilst watching for the chest to rise *(rescue breath)*. Take about one second to make the chest rise.

- Keeping the airway open, remove your mouth. Take a breath of fresh air and watch for the casualty's chest to fall as air comes out.

- Re-seal your mouth and give another rescue breath *(two in total)*.

- Return your hands without delay to the correct position on the breastbone and give another 30 chest compressions *(then 2 more rescue breaths)*.

- **Continue repeating cycles of 30 chest compressions and 2 rescue breaths.**

- Only stop to recheck the casualty if they start breathing normally – otherwise don't interrupt resuscitation.

If your rescue breaths don't make the chest rise effectively, give another 30 chest compressions, then before your next attempt:

- Check the casualty's mouth and remove any visible obstruction.

- Recheck that there is adequate head tilt and chin lift.

- Do not attempt more than two breaths each time before returning to chest compressions.

NOTE: If there is more than one rescuer, change over every two minutes to prevent fatigue. Ensure the minimum of delay as you change over.

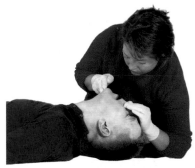

Arms straight and shoulders above your hands, depress the chest 4 to 5cm.

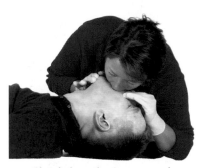

Nip the nose and seal your mouth around the casualty's mouth.

continue resuscitation until:

- Qualified help arrives and takes over.

- The casualty starts breathing normally, or

- You become exhausted.

Slowly breathe just enough air to make the chest rise.

resuscitation

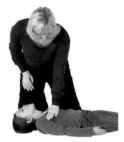

For a child over 1 year, use one or two hands to compress the chest by about one third of its depth.

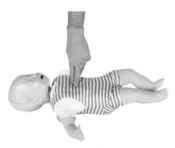

For a baby under 1 year, use two fingers to compress the chest by about one third of its depth.

resuscitation for children and babies

Recent studies have found that many children do not receive resuscitation because potential rescuers fear causing them harm. It is important to understand that it's far better to perform 'adult style' resuscitation on a child *(who is unresponsive and not breathing)* than to do nothing at all.

For ease of learning and retention, first aiders can use the adult sequence of resuscitation *(see previous pages)* on a child or baby who is unresponsive and not breathing. The following minor modifications to the adult sequence will, however, make it even more suitable for use in children:

- Give **five** initial rescue breaths before starting chest compressions *(then continue at the ratio of **30** compressions to **2** breaths).*

- If you are on your own, perform resuscitation for about 1 minute before going for help.

- Compress the chest by about one-third of its depth:

  - For a baby under 1 year, use **two fingers**.

  - For a child over 1 year, use **one or two hands** *(as needed)* to achieve an adequate depth of compression *(about one third of the depth).*

chest compression only resuscitation

When an adult casualty suffers a cardiac arrest, it is likely that there is residual oxygen left in the blood stream.

If you are unable *(or unwilling)* to give rescue breaths, give 'chest compressions only' resuscitation, as this will circulate any residual oxygen in the blood stream, so it is better than no CPR at all.

- If chest compressions only are given, these should be continuous at a rate of 100 per minute.

- Stop to recheck the casualty only if they start breathing normally – otherwise do not interrupt resuscitation.

- If there is more than one rescuer, change over every two minutes to prevent fatigue. Ensure the minimum of delay as you change over.

vomiting

It is common for a patient who has stopped breathing to vomit whilst they are collapsed. This is a passive action in the unconscious person, so you may not hear or see it happening. You might not find out until you give a rescue breath *(as the air comes back out of the patient it makes gurgling noises).*

- If the patient has vomited, turn them onto their side, tip the head back and allow the vomit to run out.

- Clean the face of the patient then continue resuscitation, using a protective face barrier if possible.

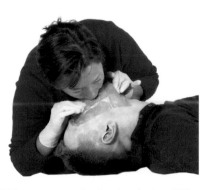

Using a protective barrier during CPR.

hygiene during resuscitation:

- Wipe the lips clean.

- If possible use a protective barrier such as a 'resusci–aid'. *(This is particularly important if the patient suffers from any serious infectious disease such as TB or S.A.R.S.).*

- As a last resort some plastic with a hole in it, or a handkerchief, may help to prevent direct contact.

- If you are still in doubt about the safety of performing rescue breaths, give 'chest compression only' resuscitation *(see above).*

- Wear protective gloves if available and wash your hands afterwards.

the main causes of unconsciousness

The causes of unconsciousness can be remembered by using 'FISH SHAPED.' Each of these causes are dealt with individually elsewhere in this manual.

Fainting

Imbalance of heat

Shock

Head Injury

Stroke

Heart Attack

Asphyxia

Poisoning

Epilepsy

Diabetes

Unconsciousness can be defined as an interruption in the normal activity of the brain. Unlike sleep, unconsciousness can disable the body's natural reflexes such as coughing. Therefore if the unconscious patient is laying on their back the tongue may fall back blocking the airway, or they may even drown themselves if they vomit.

You should take immediate action to treat an unconscious casualty. This will involve protecting the airway, calling an ambulance and possibly treating the underlying cause of the condition.

levels of response

In order to accurately measure a casualty's conscious level, we can use a scale of consciousness called the 'AVPU' scale:

Alert	**The casualty is fully alert** They are responsive and fully orientated *(a casualty in this category will usually know what month it is).*
Voice	**Confused** The casualty is not fully orientated but asks and answers your questions.
	Inappropriate Words The patient is able to speak words, but cannot put them together into logical sentences.
	Utters Sounds The casualty is not able to speak words but makes noises, often in response to painful stimuli.
	No Verbal Response The casualty makes no noise.
Pain	**Localises Pain** The patient is able to localise where painful stimuli is being applied.
	Responds to *(but does not localise)* **Pain** The patient responds to painful stimuli, but is unable to localise it.
Unresponsive	**Unresponsive** The casualty is unresponsive to pain and speech stimuli.

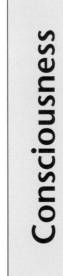

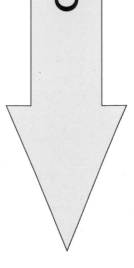

Consciousness

The Primary and Secondary Survey methods of checking a patient give us a systematic order in which to deal with the most urgent problems first, then move on to find other clues – helping with diagnosis and treatment.

primary survey

When you check for **D**anger, **R**esponse, **A**irway and **B**reathing this is called the 'Primary Survey.' This can be found in the 'resuscitation' section of this manual *(see page 6).*

The primary survey ensures that the patient is breathing, so it should be carried out first.

Once you are sure that the patient is breathing effectively, it is safe to move on and carry out a secondary survey:

secondary survey

If a casualty is unconscious you are concerned about the airway for any reason *(e.g. vomiting)*, place them in the recovery position immediately *(page 11).*

The Secondary Survey should be done quickly and systematically, first checking for major bleeding and then broken bones.

Bleeding	• Do a quick head to toe check for bleeding. • Check the hidden area such as under the arch of the back. • Control any major bleeding that you find *(page 30).*
Head and neck	• Clues to injury could be bruising, swelling, deformity or bleeding. • Check the whole head and face. • Feel the back of the neck. • Has the patient had an accident that might have injured the neck? *(page 38).*
Shoulders and chest	• Place your hands on opposite shoulders and compare them. • Run your fingers down the collar bones checking for signs of a fracture *(page 37).* • Gently squeeze and rock the ribs.
Abdomen and pelvis	• Push the abdomen with the palm of your hand to check for abnormality or response to pain. • Gently check the pelvis for signs of a fracture. • Look for incontinence or bleeding.
Legs and arms	• Feel each leg for the signs of a fracture. • Feel each arm for the signs of a fracture. • Look for other clues *(medic alert bracelets, needle marks etc).*
Pockets	• Look for clues and make sure nothing will injure the patient as you roll them into the recovery position. • Have a witness if you remove items from pockets. • Be very careful if you suspect there could be sharp objects such as needles. • Loosen any tight clothing.
Recovery	• Place the patient in the recovery position *(page 11).* • **If you suspect neck injury, get someone to help you keep the head in line with the body as you turn the patient** *(see page 40 for how to do this).* • Be careful not to cause further damage to any suspected injuries.

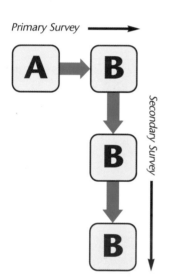

Primary Survey ⟶

A → B

Secondary Survey

B

B

Remember the priorities of treatment?
(page 4)

mechanics of injury

Before you move a patient, it is important to consider the 'mechanics of injury'.

This involves trying to work out what happened and what injuries this could have caused the patient.

- **If you suspect neck injury, get someone to help you keep the head in line with the body at all times** *(see page 40 for how to do this)*.
- If you have to use the recovery position, try not to move any suspected injuries.

the recovery position

When an unconscious person is lying on their back, there are 2 main dangers that can compromise the airway:

The Tongue: Touching the back of the throat.

Vomit: If the patient is sick *(see page 8)*.

By placing the casualty in the recovery position, the tongue won't touch the back of the throat. If the casualty is sick, the vomit will run out of the mouth and keep the airway clear.

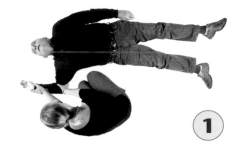

to place someone in the recovery position:

- Remove the patient's glasses.
- Kneel beside the patient and make sure that both their legs are straight.
- Make sure the airway is still open *(head tilt, chin lift)*.
- Place the arm nearest you out at right angles to the body, elbow bent with palm uppermost *(picture 1)*.
- Bring the patient's far arm across their chest, and hold the back of that hand against their cheek *(picture 2)*.
- With your other hand, grasp the far leg just above the knee, and pull it up, keeping the foot on the ground *(picture 3)*.
- Keeping their hand pressed against their cheek, pull on the leg to roll them towards you, onto their side.
- Adjust the upper leg so that both the hip and the knee are bent at right angles *(picture 4)*.
- Tilt the head back to make sure the airway remains open.
- Adjust the hand under the cheek, if necessary, to keep the head tilted.
- **Dial 999 for an ambulance if this has not already been done.**
- Check breathing regularly. Monitor the pulse in the lower arm *(radial)* if possible.
- If the patient is in the recovery position for a long period of time, turn them onto their opposite side every 30 minutes.

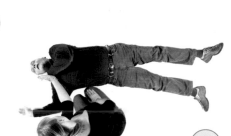

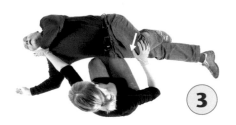

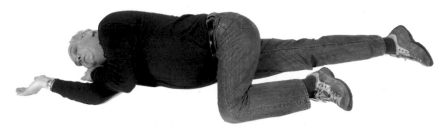

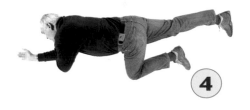

NEVER place anything in an unconscious casualty's mouth.

NEVER place a pillow under the head whilst the casualty is on their back.

NEVER move a casualty without checking them first.

NEVER move the casualty unnecessarily.

serious head injuries

Any head injury is potentially a very serious condition. Injuries to the head often lead to unconsciousness, which in turn compromises the airway. Permanent damage to the brain may result from a head injury.

It is important to remember that any patient with a head injury may also have a spinal injury to the neck *(see pages 38-40)*.

Three conditions that may be present with head injuries are concussion, compression and fractured skull:

concussion

Concussion is a condition caused by 'shaking' of the brain. The brain is cushioned within the skull by 'cerebro-spinal fluid', so if the head receives a blow the brain can bounce from one side to the other, causing widespread disruption to its normal functioning. The casualty may become unconscious for a short period *(usually less than 3 minutes)*, after which the levels of response *(see page 9)* should improve. The casualty should recover completely if no complications are present.

compression

Compression is a very serious condition, because the brain is placed under extreme pressure, caused by bleeding or swelling in the cranial cavity *(see diagram)*. The cause of compression can be from a skull fracture or head injury, but can also occur from illness, such as a ruptured blood vessel *(a type of stroke)*, a brain tumour or infection *(such as meningitis)*.

fractured skull

A skull fracture is serious because the broken bone may directly damage the brain, or cause bleeding, which in turn results in compression. Suspect a skull fracture with any patient who has received a head injury, especially if the patient has lowered levels of response *(page 9)*.

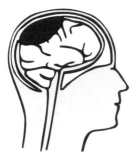

Compression – bleeding in the cranial cavity exerts pressure on the brain.

possible signs and symptoms ?

Concussion	Compression	Fractured Skull
Possibly unconscious for a short period, followed by an improvement in levels of response and recovery.	Could have a history of recent head injury with apparent recovery, but then deteriorates.	The patient may also suffer from concussion or compression, so those signs and symptoms might be present.
Short term memory loss *(particularly of the incident)*. Confusion, irritability.	Levels of response become worse as condition develops.	Bleeding, swelling or bruising of the head.
Mild, general headache.	Intense headache.	Soft area or depression on the scalp.
Pale, clammy skin.	Flushed, dry skin.	Bruising around one or both eyes.
Shallow / normal breathing.	Deep, noisy, slow breathing. *(Pressure on breathing area of the brain)*	Bruising or swelling behind an ear.
Rapid, weak pulse. *(Blood diverts away from the extremities)*	Slow, strong pulse. *(Caused by raised blood pressure)*	Bleeding or fluid coming from an ear or the nose.
Normal pupils, reacting to light.	One or both pupils may dilate as pressure increases on the brain.	Deformity or lack of symmetry to the head.
Possible nausea or vomiting on recovery.	Condition becomes worse. Fits may occur. No recovery.	Blood in the white of the eye.

treatment of serious head injury

WARNING! A patient suffering from head injury may also have a neck injury, so treat the patient with care *(see pages 38 to 40)*.

- **Dial 999 for an ambulance** if the casualty has been unconscious, their levels of response deteriorate, or you suspect fractured skull.
- Maintain **Airway** and **Breathing** *(pages 6 to 8)*.
- If the casualty is unconscious and breathing, use the jaw thrust method to keep the airway open, because this doesn't move the neck *(see page 39 and 40)*.
- If you can't keep the airway clear using the jaw thrust method, place the patient in the recovery position. Keep the head, neck and body in line as you turn the patient *(see page 40)*.
- If the casualty is conscious, help them to lie down. Keep the head, neck and body in line in case there is a neck injury.
- Control any bleeding by applying gentle pressure around the wound, but if there is bleeding or discharge from an ear, don't try to plug the ear or stop it bleeding.
- Look for and treat any other injuries.

useful tips for head injury treatment:

- Constantly monitor and record breathing, pulse and the levels of response. Even if the casualty appears to recover, watch out for a subsequent reduction in levels of response *(page 9)*.
- Make sure that a concussed casualty who recovers is not alone for the next few hours. Advise them to see a doctor as soon as possible.
- Advise the patient to go to hospital immediately if they suffer from headache, nausea, vomiting or excessive sleepiness in the next few days.
- Don't allow a concussed sports player to 'play on' until they have seen a doctor.

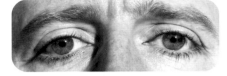

Pinpoint pupils

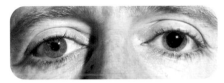

Unequal pupils

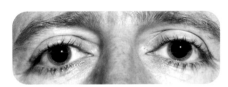

Dilated pupils

stroke

The clinical name for stroke is 'cerebro-vascular accident' (CVA).

60% of strokes are caused by a blood clot (thrombosis) in an artery supplying the brain. Most of the patients who suffer this type of stroke are elderly people. The other form of stroke is caused by bleeding into the cranial cavity following the rupture of an artery. Patients who suffer this type of stroke can be younger, and often have a history of high blood pressure.

possible signs and symptoms ?

- Weakness or paralysis down one side of the body or face.
- Slurred or confused speech.
- Gradual or sudden loss of consciousness.
- Unequal pupil size *(see pictures)*.
- Agitation or aggression to the point of crying.
- Headache.
- Slow, strong pulse.
- Slow, deep, noisy breathing.
- Flushed, dry skin.
- Vomiting or incontinence.

treatment of stroke

- Maintain **Airway** and **Breathing** *(page 6 to 8)*.
- **Dial 999 for an ambulance.**
- Place an unconscious casualty in the recovery position.
- Lay the conscious casualty down, with head and shoulders raised.
- Reassure the casualty – do not assume that they don't understand.
- Monitor and record breathing, pulse and levels of response.

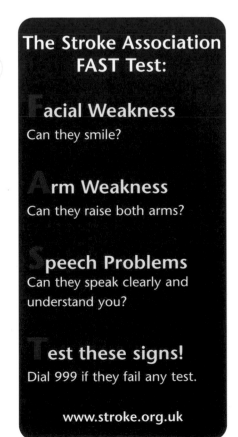

The Stroke Association FAST Test:

Facial Weakness
Can they smile?

Arm Weakness
Can they raise both arms?

Speech Problems
Can they speak clearly and understand you?

Test these signs!
Dial 999 if they fail any test.

www.stroke.org.uk

unconsciousness

hypoxia

The medical term 'hypoxia' means 'low oxygen in the blood'.

A low level of oxygen in the blood is potentially fatal, so it is very important that the First Aider recognises the signs and symptoms of this condition and takes immediate action to treat the casualty.

The causes of hypoxia can be separated into 5 areas:

possible signs and symptoms ?

- *Pale clammy skin.*
- *Blue tinges to the skin (cyanosis).*
- *Increase in pulse rate.*
- *Weakening of the pulse.*
- *Nausea or vomiting.*
- *Increased breathing rate (caused by oxygen deficiency).*
- *Lowered breathing rate (look for control centre causes).*
- *Distressed breathing or gasping.*
- *Confusion or dizziness.*
- *Lowering levels of consciousness.*
- *Clues from the cause of the hypoxia (i.e. bleeding, injury, chest pain etc).*

external causes:

Not enough oxygen in the surrounding air, such as:

- Suffocation by gas or smoke.
- Drowning.
- Suffocation by sand, earth or a pillow etc.
- High altitude.

airway causes:

Blockage, swelling or narrowing. Caused by:

- The tongue.
- Vomit.
- Choking.
- Burns.
- Strangulation.
- Hanging.
- Anaphylaxis.

breathing causes:

Inability of the lungs to function properly. Caused by:

- Crushing of the chest.
- Collapsed lung.
- Chest injury.
- Poisoning.
- Asthma.
- Disease or illness.

circulation causes:

Inability of the blood to take up oxygen, a fall in blood pressure, or failure to circulate the blood around the body. Caused by:

- Heart attack.
- Cardiac arrest.
- Angina.
- Severe bleeding.
- Poisoning.
- Anaemia.

control centre causes:

Failure of the respiratory control centre in the brain or the nerves connecting it to the lungs. Caused by:

- Stroke.
- Head injury.
- Drug overdose.
- Poisoning.
- Spinal injury.
- Electric shock.

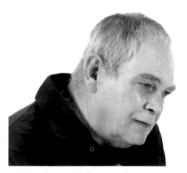

Pale clammy skin and cyanosis.

treatment of hypoxia ✚

- *Maintain **Airway** and **Breathing** (pages 6 to 8).*
- *Remove or treat the **cause** of the hypoxia.*
- *Do not allow the patient to eat, drink or smoke.*

the body's response to hypoxia

If the body detects low levels of oxygen in the blood ADRENALINE is released. The effect of adrenaline on the body is to:

- Increase the heart rate.
- Increase the strength of the heart beat *(and blood pressure)*.
- Divert blood away from the skin, intestines and stomach.
- Divert blood towards the heart, lungs and brain.
- Dilate the air passages in the lungs *(bronchioles)*.

The effect of adrenaline being released in the body produces dramatic signs and symptoms that the first aider must be able to recognise.

Can you tell which of the signs and symptoms are caused by adrenaline?

the respiratory system

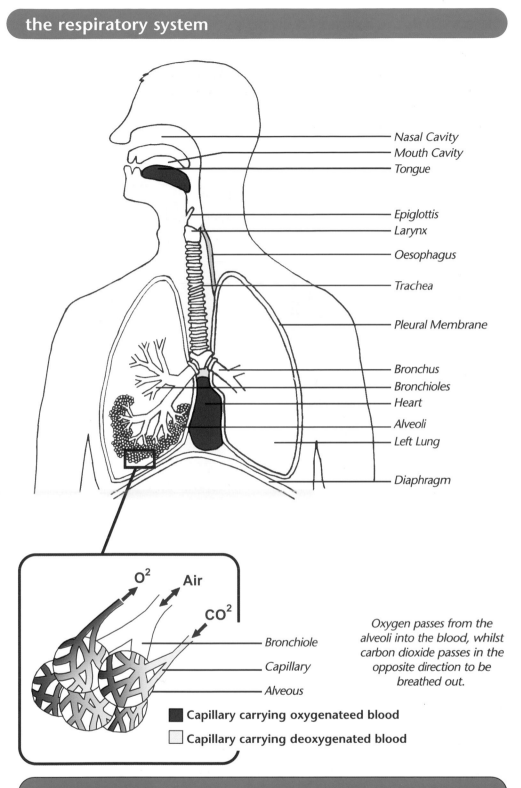

Nasal Cavity
Mouth Cavity
Tongue
Epiglottis
Larynx
Oesophagus
Trachea
Pleural Membrane
Bronchus
Bronchioles
Heart
Alveoli
Left Lung
Diaphragm

O^2 Air
CO^2

Bronchiole
Capillary
Alveous

■ Capillary carrying oxygenateed blood
□ Capillary carrying deoxygenated blood

Oxygen passes from the alveoli into the blood, whilst carbon dioxide passes in the opposite direction to be breathed out.

Air is drawn in through the mouth and nose, where it is warmed, filtered and moistened.

Air then travels through the throat and past the epiglottis (the protective flap of skin that folds down to protect the airway when we swallow).

Air now enters the larynx (more commonly known as the voice box or 'Adam's apple'). It passes between the vocal cords in the larynx and down into the trachea.

The trachea is protected by rings of cartilage that surround it to prevent kinking.

The trachea divides into two 'bronchi' that supply air to each lung.

The bronchi then divide into smaller air passages called 'bronchioles'.

At the end of the bronchioles are microscopic air sacks called 'alveoli'.

The walls of the alveoli are only one cell in thickness, so oxygen can pass through into the blood, which is carried in capillaries that surround the alveoli.

Carbon dioxide (a waste gas from the body) passes from the blood into the alveoli, and is then breathed out.

The trachea, bronchi, and lungs are contained in the 'thoracic cavity' in the chest.

To draw air down into the thoracic cavity, the diaphragm flattens and the chest walls move out. This increases the size of the thoracic cavity, creating a negative pressure which draws air in.

Each lung is surrounded by a two layered membrane called the 'pleura'.

Between the two layers of the pleura is a thin layer of 'serous' fluid, which enables the chest walls to move freely.

The thoracic cavity is protected by the ribs, which curl around from the spine and connect to the sternum (breast bone) at the front of the body.

What's in the air that we breathe?

Air that we breathe in:		Air that we breathe out:	
Oxygen	20%	Oxygen	16%
Carbon Dioxide	Trace	Carbon Dioxide	4%
Nitrogen	79%	Nitrogen	79%
Other Gases	1%	Other Gases	1%

'Normal' Respiratory Rates

Adult	12 - 20 breaths / minute
Child	20 - 40 breaths / minute
Baby	30 - 60 breaths / minute

airway and breathing problems

choking

One of the most successful skills that can be learned by the first aider is the treatment of a casualty who is choking. Objects such as food, sweets or small objects can easily become lodged in the airway if they are accidentally 'breathed in' rather than swallowed.

possible signs and symptoms

- The patient is unable to speak or cough.
- Grasping or pointing to the throat.
- Distressed look on the face.
- Congestion of the face initially.
- Pale skin and cyanosis in later stages.
- Unconsciousness in later stages.

choking adult or child *(over 1 year)*

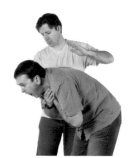

Back slaps.

Firstly, encourage the patient to cough. If the choking is only mild, this will clear the obstruction and the patient should be able to speak to you.

If the obstruction is not cleared:

1   back slaps

- **Shout for help**, but don't leave the patient yet.
- Bend the casualty forwards so the head is lower than the chest. For a smaller child you can place them over your knee to do this.
- Give up to 5 firm blows between the shoulder blades with the palm of your hand. Check between blows and stop if you clear the obstruction.

If the obstruction is still not cleared:

2   abdominal thrusts

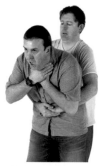

Abdominal thrusts.

- Stand behind the casualty *(or kneel behind a small child)*. Place both your arms around their waist.
- Make a fist with one hand and place it just above the belly button *(below the ribs)* with your thumb inwards.
- Grasp this fist with your other hand, then pull sharply inwards and upwards. Do this up to 5 times. Check between thrusts and stop if you clear the obstruction.

If the obstruction is still not cleared:

3   repeat steps 1 and 2

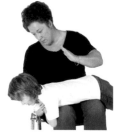

Back slaps performed on a smaller child.

- Keep repeating steps 1 and 2.
- If the treatment seems ineffective, shout for help. Ask someone to **dial 999 for an ambulance**, but don't interrupt the treatment whilst the patient is still conscious.

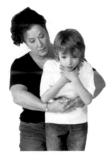

Abdominal thrusts performed on a smaller child.

> *Abdominal thrusts can cause serious internal injuries, so send the patient to see a doctor.*
> *After successful treatment, patients with a persistent cough, difficulty swallowing or with the feeling of an 'object still stuck in the throat' should also see a doctor.*

choking – baby *(under 1 year)*

The baby may attempt to cough. If the choking is only mild, this will clear the obstruction – the baby may cry and should now be able to breathe effectively.

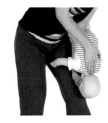

Abdominal thrusts should **NOT** be performed on a baby

If the obstruction is not cleared:

1 back slaps

- **Shout for help**, but don't leave the baby yet.
- Lay the baby over your arm, face down, legs either side of your elbow with the head below the chest *(see diagram)*.
- Give up to 5 blows between the shoulder blades with the palms of your fingers. Check between blows and stop if you clear the obstruction.

If the obstruction is still not cleared:

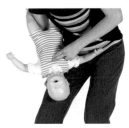

Back slaps.

2 chest thrusts

- Turn the baby over, chest uppermost *(by laying them on your other arm)* and lower the head below the level of the chest.
- Using two fingers on the chest, give up to 5 chest thrusts. These are similar to chest compressions, but sharper in nature and delivered at a slower rate. Check between thrusts and stop if you clear the obstruction.

If the obstruction is still not cleared:

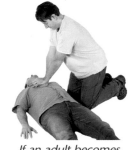

Chest thrusts.

3 repeat steps 1 and 2

- Keep repeating steps 1 and 2.
- If the treatment seems ineffective, shout for help. Ask someone to **dial 999 for an ambulance**, but don't interrupt the treatment yet.

if an ADULT becomes unconscious:

- Support the casualty carefully to the ground and immediately **dial 999 for an ambulance** *(if not already done)*.
- Start CPR – follow the sequence on page 7 after the heading 'if the casualty is not breathing normally:'

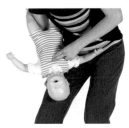

If an adult becomes unconscious – start CPR.

if a CHILD or BABY becomes unconscious:

Place the child or baby on a firm, flat surface and start CPR as follows:

- Open the airway and check in the mouth. Pick out any visible obstruction *(but don't try to reach blindly into the back of the throat)*.
- Attempt 5 rescue breaths. **If there is no response**:
  - Immediately give 30 chest compressions *(even if your breaths were successful)*.
  - Repeat cycles of 2 rescue breaths then 30 compressions.
- Check the mouth each time before you give rescue breaths. Pick out any visible obstruction *(but don't try to reach blindly into the back of the throat)*.
- If you are on your own, give CPR for 1 minute then **dial 999 for an ambulance** *(if not already done)*.
- Continue CPR until the child starts breathing normally on its own, help arrives to take over, or you become exhausted.

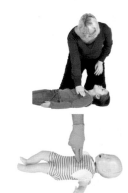

If a child or baby becomes unconscious – attempt 5 rescue breaths then start CPR.

anaphylaxis

Anaphylaxis is an extremely dangerous allergic reaction. The name 'anaphylaxis' means 'without protection' and indeed, the condition is caused by a massive over-reaction of the body's protection *(immune)* system.

Anaphylaxis is very rare. The most common reactions are to drugs *(such as penicillin)*. Other common allergies are to things such as insect stings, peanuts, seafoods etc.

The main chemical that the immune cells release if they detect a 'foreign protein' is **_histamine_**. Histamine has several effects on the body when it is released in massive quantities:

- It makes blood vessels dilate.
- It constricts the bronchioles in the lungs.
- It makes blood capillary walls 'leaky', causing severe swelling and shock *(page 26)*.
- It weakens the strength of the heart's contractions.
- It makes the skin itchy.
- It makes the skin come out in a rash.

possible signs and symptoms ?

The allergic reaction can happen in seconds, so fast recognition is essential:

- Sudden swelling of the face, tongue, lips, neck and eyes.
- Hoarse voice, 'lump in the throat', developing into loud pitched noisy breathing *(which may stop altogether)*.
- Difficult, wheezy breathing, tight chest *(the patient may have the equivalent of an asthma attack as well as a swollen airway)*.
- Rapid weak pulse.
- Nausea, vomiting, stomach cramps, diarrhoea.
- Itchy skin.
- Red, blotchy skin eruption.
- Anxiety – a feeling of 'impending doom'.

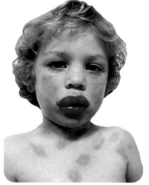

This child has swelling of the tongue and lips and a red blotchy rash on his chest.

treatment

- **Dial 999 for an ambulance.**
- Help the conscious casualty to sit up to help breathing.
- If the casualty becomes unconscious – lay them down then check **Airway** and **Breathing** *(pages 6 to 8)*.
- Resuscitate as necessary.

NOTE: A patient who has suffered a previous anaphylactic reaction may carry a syringe of adrenaline (two common brand names are 'Epi–Pen' and 'Ana-Pen').

This can save the casualty's life if it's given promptly. The patient should be able to inject this on their own but, if necessary, assist them to use it.

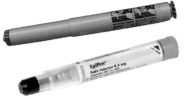

asthma

Asthma is a condition caused by an allergic reaction in the lungs, often to substances such as dust, traffic fumes, or pollen. Muscles surrounding the bronchioles *(see page 15)* go into spasm and constrict, making it very difficult for the patient to breathe.

Most asthma patients carry medication around with them, usually in the form of an inhaler. Ask the patient, but usually the **blue** inhaler is for relieving an attack, dilating the bronchioles to relieve the condition.

An asthma attack is a traumatic experience for the patient, especially a child, so reassurance and a calm approach from the First Aider is essential. If the patient is not reassured and calmed down by the First Aider, an attack can lead on to 'hyperventilation' *(see page 20)* after the inhaler has relieved the constricted airways.

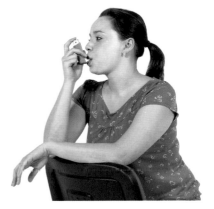

An upright sitting position usually helps the patient to breathe more easily. Help the patient to take their own inhaler (the blue one is for relieving the attack).

possible signs and symptoms   **?**

- Difficulty breathing.
- Wheezy breath sounds, originating from the lungs.
- Difficulty speaking *(will need to take a breath in the middle of a sentence)*.
- Pale, clammy skin.
- Grey or blue lips and skin *(cyanosis)*.
- Use of muscles in the neck and upper chest to help the casualty breathe.
- Casualty will become exhausted in a severe attack.
- May become unconscious and stop breathing in a prolonged attack.

treatment of asthma attack   ✚

- Keep calm and be reassuring towards the casualty.
- Help the casualty to sit upright, leaning on a table or chair if necessary.
- Help the casualty to take their own medication.
- Try to take the casualty's mind off the attack – make conversation.
- If the attack is prolonged, the patient appears to be in severe respiratory distress, or the medication is not effective, **dial 999 for an ambulance**.
- Do not take the casualty into the cold winter air.
- Keep the casualty upright – even if they become too weak to sit up on their own. Only lay an asthma attack patient down if they become unconscious.
- Be prepared to carry out resuscitation *(page 6 to 8)*.

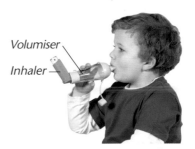

Volumiser

Inhaler

Some asthma patients need to use a 'volumiser' because they can't take their inhaler all in one breath.

croup

Croup is a condition usually suffered by very young children, where the larynx and trachea become infected and swollen. The attacks, which often occur during the night, can appear very alarming, but nearly always clear without causing the child any lasting harm.

possible signs and symptoms   **?**

- Difficult distressed breathing.
- A loud pitched, or whistling noise as the child breathes.
- A short 'barking' type cough.
- Pale, clammy skin.
- Blue tinges to the skin *(cyanosis)*.
- Use of muscles in the neck and upper chest to help the child breathe.

treatment of croup   ✚

- Keep calm – panic will distress the child and make the attack worse.
- Sit the child up and reassure them.
- Create a steamy atmosphere in the room – boil a kettle, run a hot bath or the shower. Beware, hot water and steam can burn.
- If the condition eases, keep the room where the child rests humid. This may prevent a further attack. Stay with the child all night.
- Call the doctor. If the attack is severe, does not ease, or the child has a temperature, **dial 999 for an ambulance**.

NEVER put your fingers down the throat of a child that appears to be suffering from croup. There is a small chance that the condition could be 'epiglottitis'. If this is the case, the epiglottis may swell even more, totally blocking the airway.

airway and breathing problems

"The contrasting difference between asthma and hyperventilation is the large volumes of air that can be heard entering the lungs of the hyperventilating patient, compared with the tight wheeze of the asthmatic"

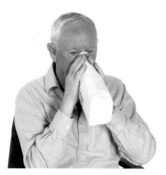

One of the possible treatments for hyperventilation (see note, below)

NOTE: *Only use the paper bag treatment if other attempts to calm the breathing have failed. Ask the patient to breathe slowly in and out of the bag for 10 breaths, then without it for 5 breaths. Repeat this cycle until the patient is able to breathe normally.*

DO NOT *use a paper bag if the patient shows any signs of hypoxia (page 14).*

hyperventilation

'Hyperventilation' means 'excessive breathing'. When we breathe in, there is only a trace of carbon dioxide in the air. When we breathe out, we breathe out 4% carbon dioxide. Hyperventilating results in low levels of carbon dioxide in the blood, which causes the signs and symptoms of this condition.

A hyperventilation attack can often result from the patient being very anxious, from a panic attack or sudden fright. The condition of hyperventilation is often mistaken for 'asthma'. Asthmatics may hyperventilate after their inhalers have taken effect *(opening the airways)*. The contrasting difference in the two conditions is the large volumes of air that can be heard entering the lungs of the hyperventilating patient, compared with the tight wheeze of the asthmatic.

possible signs and symptoms

- Unnaturally deep, fast breathing.
- Attention seeking behaviour.
- Dizziness, faintness.
- Feeling of a 'tight' chest.
- Cramps in the hands and feet.
- Flushed skin, **no cyanosis.**
- Pins and needles in the arms and hands.
- The patient may think they cannot breathe.
- If the attack is prolonged, the casualty may pass out and stop breathing for up to 30 seconds.

treatment of hyperventilation

- Be firm and calm, but reassuring with the casualty.
- Move them to a quiet place with few people around.
- Explain to the casualty that they are hyperventilating.
- 'Coach' the casualty's breathing.
- Asking the patient to take tiny sips of water will reduce the number of breaths they can take.
- Breathing through the nose or into a paper bag will reduce the loss of carbon dioxide, but the casualty will need lots of reassurance *(see note, left)*.
- Call for medical advice if the attack is prolonged or you are in doubt.

drowning

Contrary to popular opinion, a casualty who drowns does not usually inhale large amounts of water into the lungs. 90% of deaths from drowning are caused by a relatively small amount of water entering the lungs, interfering with oxygen exchange in the alveoli *(wet drowning)*. The other 10% are caused by muscle spasm near the epiglottis and larynx blocking the airway *(dry drowning)*. The casualty will usually **swallow** large amounts of water, which might then be vomited as they are rescued or resuscitation takes place.

It should be remembered that other factors may contribute to the cause of drowning – for example hypothermia, alcohol, or an underlying medical condition such as epilepsy or heart attack.

secondary drowning

If a small amount of water enters the lungs, irritation is caused and fluid is drawn from the blood into the alveoli. This reaction could be delayed for several hours, so a casualty who has been resuscitated and 'apparently recovered' might relapse into severe difficulty breathing at a later stage. It is for this reason that any casualty who recovers from 'near drowning' should be taken to hospital immediately.

NEVER *enter the water to rescue a drowning casualty unless you have been trained to do so. Try to reach them with a rope or stick, or throw them an object that will float. "Reach or throw – don't GO"*

treatment of drowning

- Do not put yourself at risk. **'Reach or throw – don't GO'.**
- If possible keep the casualty horizontal during rescue, as shock can occur.
- Check **Airway** and **Breathing**. – Perform CPR if necessary *(page 6 to 8)*.
- **Dial 999 for an ambulance,** even if the casualty appears to recover.

collapsed lung / sucking chest wound

Each lung is surrounded by 2 layers of membrane called the 'pleura'. Between these 2 membranes is the 'pleural cavity', containing a very thin layer of 'serous fluid', which enables the two layers to move against each other as we breathe.

In a penetrating chest injury, where the outer layer of the pleura is damaged, air can be sucked from the outside of the chest into the pleural cavity, causing the lung to collapse (pneumothorax).

In any serious chest injury, the inner layer of the pleura could become perforated. Air may then be drawn from the lung into the pleural cavity, again causing the lung to collapse.

If air continues to be sucked into the pleural cavity, but cannot escape, pressure in the collapsed lung can build (tension pneumothorax). This pressure build up can squeeze the heart and the uninjured lung, making it difficult for both to function.

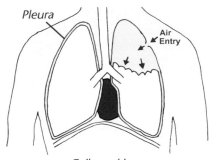

Pleura

Air Entry

Collapsed lung.

possible signs and symptoms ?

- Severe difficulty breathing.
- Painful breathing.
- Fast, shallow breathing.
- Cyanosis of lips and skin.
- Pale, clammy skin.
- Uneven chest movements – the injured side of the chest may not rise.

If there is a sucking chest wound:

- Sound of air being drawn into the wound, with bubbling blood.
- Crackling feeling of the skin around the injury *(because of air entry)*.

treatment ✚

- Immediately cover a sucking chest wound with your hand *(or the casualty's hand if they are conscious)* to prevent air entry.
- **Dial 999 for an ambulance** – send someone to do this if possible.
- Place a sterile pad over the wound, then cover it with plastic, cling film, kitchen foil or other air tight covering.
- Tape the air tight covering on 3 sides. The dressing should prevent air from entering the wound, but still allow air to get out.
- If the casualty becomes unconscious: open the **Airway**, check **Breathing** and resuscitate if necessary. Place them in the recovery position with the injured side lowest. This will help to protect the uninjured lung.

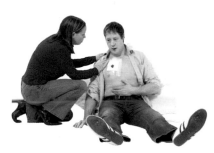

Tape the air tight covering on 3 sides. The dressing should prevent air from entering the wound, but still allow air to get out.

flail chest

This is a condition where the ribs surrounding the chest have become fractured in several places, creating a 'floating' section of the chest wall.

As the casualty breathes, the rest of the chest wall moves out, but the flail segment moves inwards. As the chest wall moves back in, the flail segment moves outwards. These are called 'paradoxical' chest movements.

possible signs and symptoms ?

- Severe difficulty breathing.
- Shallow, painful breathing.
- Signs and symptoms of a fracture *(page 37)*.
- 'Paradoxical' chest movements *(see above)*.

treatment ✚

- **Dial 999 for an ambulance.**
- Place the casualty in the position they find most comfortable – sat up, inclined towards the injury if possible.
- Place large amounts of padding over the flail area.
- Place the arm on the injured side in an elevated sling. Squeeze the arm gently against the padding to provide gentle, firm support to the injury.

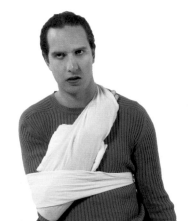

Place padding over the flail area and place the arm on the injured side in an elevated sling.

circulation problems

the circulatory system

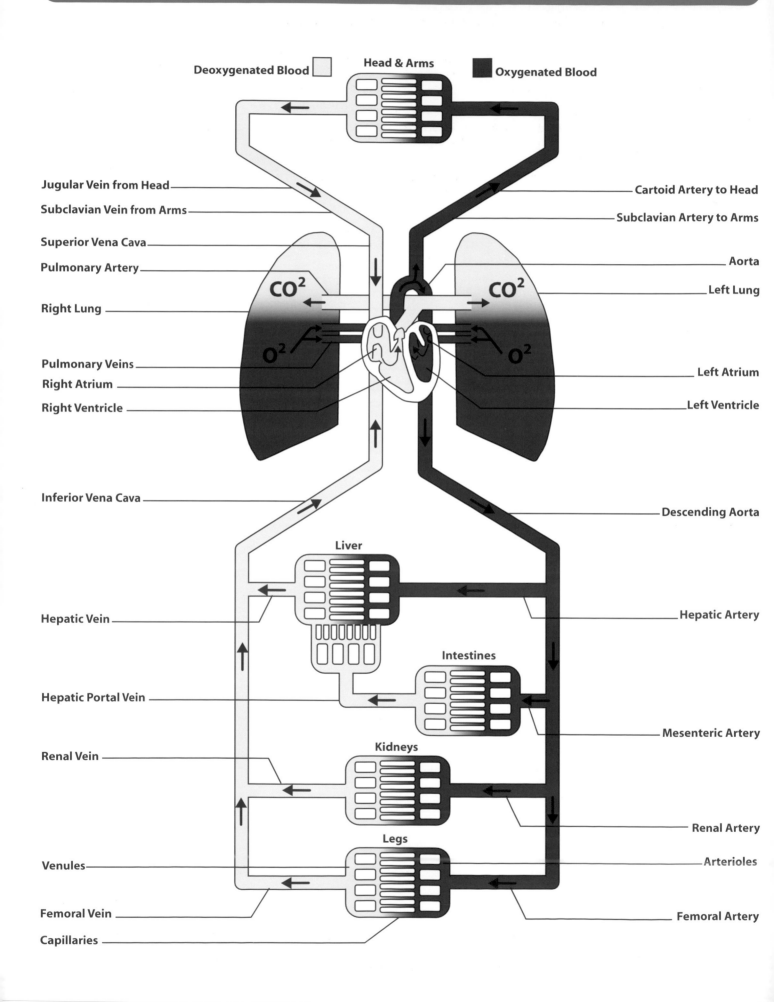

Deoxygenated Blood

Head & Arms

Oxygenated Blood

Jugular Vein from Head

Subclavian Vein from Arms

Superior Vena Cava

Pulmonary Artery

CO^2

CO^2

Right Lung

O^2

O^2

Pulmonary Veins

Right Atrium

Right Ventricle

Cartoid Artery to Head

Subclavian Artery to Arms

Aorta

Left Lung

Left Atrium

Left Ventricle

Inferior Vena Cava

Descending Aorta

Liver

Hepatic Vein

Hepatic Artery

Intestines

Hepatic Portal Vein

Mesenteric Artery

Kidneys

Renal Vein

Legs

Renal Artery

Venules

Arterioles

Femoral Vein

Femoral Artery

Capillaries

the circulatory system

The circulatory system consists of a closed network of tubes *(arteries, veins and capillaries)* connected to a pump *(the heart)*.

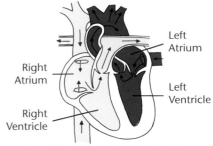

How blood flows though the four chambers of the heart.

Arteries — Carry blood **away** from the heart. They have strong, elastic, muscular walls which are able to expand as blood from the heart beating surges through. The largest artery, which connects directly to the heart, is called the 'aorta'.

Veins — Carry blood **towards** the heart. They have thinner walls than arteries because the blood in them is under less pressure. They have one-way valves, which keep blood flowing towards the heart. The largest veins, which connect to the heart, are called 'vena cava'.

Capillaries — Are the tiny blood vessels between the arteries and veins which allow the transfer of oxygen, carbon dioxide and nutrients in and out of the cells of the body.

The Heart — Is a four-chambered pump. The left and right sides of the heart are separate. The **left** side takes blood from the lungs and pumps it around the **body**. The **right** side takes blood from the body and pumps it to the **lungs**.

The two sides of the heart are separated into two chambers called the 'atria' and the 'ventricles'. The **atria** are the top chambers which **collect blood** as it returns from the lungs and the body and pump it to the ventricles. The **ventricles** then pump the blood **out of the heart**, to the lungs and around the body.

the blood

60% of the blood consists of a clear yellow fluid called plasma. Suspended within the plasma are red blood cells, white blood cells, platelets and nutrients.

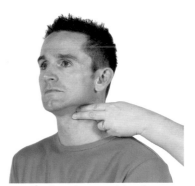

Feeling the carotid pulse.

Red Cells — Contain haemoglobin, which carries oxygen for use by the cells of the body. Red cells give the blood its colour.

White Cells — Fight infection.

Platelets — Trigger a complicated chemical reaction if a blood vessel is damaged, forming a clot.

Nutrients — Are derived from the food by the digestive system. When combined with oxygen in the cells of the body, they provide vital energy, keeping the cell alive.

- The blood carries carbon dioxide *(the waste gas produced by the cells)* mainly in the form of 'carbonic acid'. Carbonic acid is diluted within the plasma.

- The blood also circulates heat *(generated mostly by the liver)* around the body. Heat is carried to the skin by the blood if the body needs to be cooled.

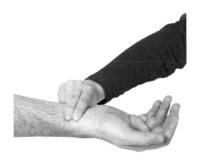

Feeling the radial pulse.

the pulse

Every time the heart contracts a pulsation of blood is pumped through the arteries. The walls of the arteries are elastic and expand as the blood flows rhythmically through. This expansion can be felt at the points where arteries come close to the skin.

When checking a pulse use the pads of the fingers, not the thumb *(which has its own pulse)*. The First Aider should make a note of the following:

Rate — Is it fast or slow? How many beats are there per minute?

Rhythm — Are the beats regular? Are there any 'missed' beats?

Strength — Does the pulse feel strong or weak?

The main pulse locations for first aid use are in the neck *(carotid pulse)*, the wrist *(radial pulse)* and the upper arm *(brachial pulse)*.

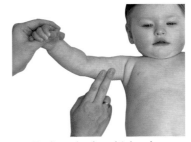

Feeling the brachial pulse on a baby.

capillary refill

Circulation to the end of an arm or leg can be checked by squeezing the tip of a finger or toe. The skin will become pale when it is squeezed – if the circulation is effective, the colour should return within 2 seconds of releasing it *(this may take longer if the hands or feet are cold)*.

'Normal' Heart Rates at Rest	
Adult	**60 - 90** beats / minute
Child	**90 - 110** beats / minute
Baby	**110 - 140** beats / minute

angina

Angina *(angina pectoris)* is a condition usually caused by the build up of a cholesterol plaque on the inner lining of a coronary artery. Cholesterol is a fatty chemical which is part of the outer lining of cells in the body. A cholesterol plaque is a hard, thick substance caused by deposits of cholesterol on the artery wall. Over time, the build up of the plaque causes narrowing and hardening of the artery.

During exercise or excitement, the heart requires more oxygen, but the narrowed coronary artery cannot increase the blood supply to meet this demand. As a result an area of the heart will suffer from a lack of oxygen. The patient will feel pain in the chest *(amongst other symptoms)* as a result.

Typically, an angina attack occurs with exertion, and subsides with rest. If the narrowing of the artery reaches a critical level, angina at rest *(called 'unstable angina')* may result. A patient with angina, especially 'unstable' angina has a high risk of suffering a heart attack in the near future.

heart attack

Heart attack *(myocardial infarction)* is often caused when the surface of a cholesterol plaque in a coronary artery cracks and has a 'rough surface'. This can lead to the formation of a blood clot on the plaque, which completely blocks the artery resulting in the death of an area of the heart muscle.

Unlike angina, the death of the heart muscle from heart attack is permanent and will not be relieved by rest.

possible signs and symptoms

It should be remembered that every heart attack is different. Only a few of the signs and symptoms may be present, indeed up to a quarter of heart attacks suffered are 'silent' *without any chest pain.*

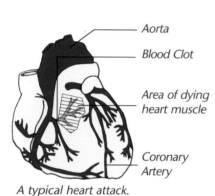

Aorta
Blood Clot
Area of dying heart muscle
Coronary Artery

A typical heart attack.

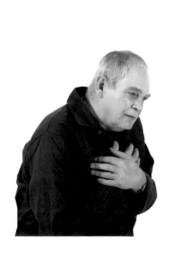

	Angina	Heart Attack
Onset	Sudden, usually during exertion, stress or extreme weather.	Sudden, can occur at rest.
Pain	'Vicelike' squashing pain, often described as 'dull', 'tightness' or 'pressure' on the chest. Can be mistaken for indigestion.	'Vicelike' squashing pain, often described as 'dull', 'tightness' or 'pressure' on the chest. Can be mistaken for indigestion.
Location of Pain	Central chest area. Can radiate into either arm *(more commonly the left)*, the neck, jaw, back, or shoulders.	Central chest area. Can radiate into either arm *(more commonly the left)*, the neck, jaw, back, or shoulders.
Duration	Usually lasts 3 to 8 minutes rarely longer.	Usually lasts longer than 30 minutes.
Skin	Pale, may be sweaty.	Pale, grey colour. May sweat profusely.
Pulse	Variable, depending on which area has a lack of oxygen. Often becomes irregular, missing beats.	Variable, depending on which area has a lack of oxygen. Often becomes irregular, missing beats.
Other Signs and Symptoms	Shortness of breath, weakness, anxiety.	Shortness of breath, dizziness, nausea, vomiting. Sense of 'impending doom'.
Factors Giving Relief	Resting, reducing stress, taking 'nitro-glycerin' medication.	Nitro-glycerin medication may give partial or no relief.

treatment of angina and heart attack

- Sit the casualty down and make them comfortable. Do not allow them to walk around. A half sitting position is often the best.

- Allow the casualty to take their own glyceryl tri-nitrate *(G.T.N.)* medication if they have it.

- Reassure the casualty. Remove any cause of stress or anxiety if possible.

- If you suspect heart attack – check the casualty is not allergic to aspirin, then allow them to **chew** an aspirin tablet **slowly**. Record the time taken and strength of the tablet. Pass this information to the paramedics or doctor.

NOTE: Aspirin reduces the clotting ability of the blood. Chewing the tablet allows the drug to absorb quickly into the blood through the skin of the mouth, so it works faster. The ideal dose is a 300mg aspirin, but any strength will do.

If you don't have any aspirin or you are not sure if you should give it, wait for the ambulance to arrive (see note, below right).

- Monitor pulse and breathing. Be prepared to resuscitate if necessary.

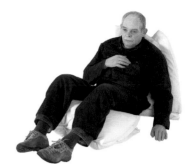

A half sitting position is often the best.

Dial 999 for an ambulance if:

- You suspect a heart attack.

- The casualty has not been diagnosed as having angina.

- The symptoms are different, or worse than the patients' normal angina attacks.

- Angina pain is not relieved by the patients' medication and rest after 15 minutes.

- You are in any doubt.

NOTE: A first aider is not allowed to 'prescribe' drugs to a patient. A fully conscious adult casualty is, however, more than capable of deciding whether or not they want to take medication that may help them.

left ventricular failure

Left ventricular failure *(LVF)* is a condition where the left ventricle of the heart *(see page 23)* is not powerful enough to empty itself. The right chamber of the heart is still working properly and pumping blood into the lungs. This results in a 'back pressure' of blood in the pulmonary veins and arteries of the lungs. Fluid from this back pressure of blood seeps into the alveoli *(see page 15)* causing *severe difficulty in breathing.*

The condition can be caused by heart attack, chronic heart failure or high blood pressure. Patients with chronic heart failure often suffer attacks during the night.

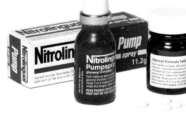

Typical G.T.N. medication that an angina patient may carry.

possible signs and symptoms ?

- Severe difficulty in breathing.

- Crackly, often wheezy breathing *(fluid on in the lungs).*

- Pale sweaty skin.

- Cyanosis *(blue grey tinges to skin and lips).*

- Coughing frothy, blood stained sputum.

- Possibility of the signs and symptoms of heart attack.

- The patient needs to sit up to breathe.

- Anxiety, confusion, dizziness.

treatment

- Sit the patient up, feet dangling.

- **Dial 999 for an ambulance.**

- Allow the patient to take their own glyceryl tri-nitrate *(G.T.N.)* medication if they have it.

- Be prepared to resuscitate – the condition can quickly deteriorate.

circulation problems

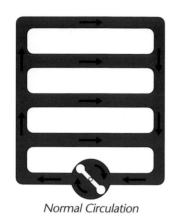

Normal Circulation

shock

To most people the word shock means an unpleasant surprise, an earthquake, or what happens if you mess about with the electrics!

The medical term shock is defined as *'inadequate tissue perfusion, caused by a fall in blood pressure or blood volume.'*

'Inadequate tissue perfusion' means an inadequate supply of oxygenated blood to the tissues of the body.

Now that you understand what shock is, you can understand why it can quickly result in death if not treated.

The more common causes of 'life threatening' shock are:

- **Hypovolaemic Shock**
- **Cardiogenic Shock**
- **Anaphylactic Shock**

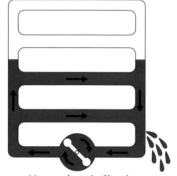

Hypovolaemic Shock

hypovolaemic shock

Hypo means **low**   *vol* means **volume**   *aemic* means **blood**

This type of shock is caused by loss of body fluids, which results in a low volume of blood.

Typical causes of hypovolaemic shock are:

- External bleeding *(pages 29 and 30).*
- Internal bleeding *(page 31).*
- Burns *(pages 33 and 34).*
- Vomiting and diarrhoea *(loss of body fluids).*
- Excessive sweating.

possible signs and symptoms *(see also blood loss: page 29)*

The first response is release of adrenaline – this will cause:

- A rise in pulse rate.
- Pale, clammy skin.

As the condition worsens:

- Fast, shallow breathing.
- Nausea or vomiting.
- Rapid, weak pulse.
- Dizziness, weakness.
- Cyanosis *(grey blue tinges to skin and lips).*
- Sweating.

As the brain suffers a lack of oxygen:

- Deep, sighing breathing *(air hunger).*
- Unconsciousness.
- Confusion, anxiety, even aggression.

treatment

- Treat the cause of the shock *(e.g. external bleeding).*
- Lay the casualty down and raise their legs in the air, returning blood to the vital organs *(take care if you suspect a fracture).*
- **Dial 999 for an ambulance.**
- Keep the casualty warm. Use coats and blankets – place a blanket under the patient if they are on a cold surface. *(Do not use hot water bottles or direct heat – this will dilate blood vessels causing the blood pressure to fall even more).*
- Loosen tight clothing around the neck, chest or waist.
- Monitor breathing, pulse and levels of response.
- Be prepared to resuscitate.

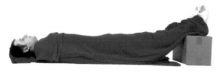

Lay the casualty down and raise the legs in the air.

cardiogenic shock

This is a fall in the blood pressure, caused by the heart not pumping effectively. This is the most common type of shock.

Typical causes of cardiogenic shock are:

- Heart attack *(page 24)*.
- Cardiac failure *(page 25)*.
- Heart valve disease.

- Tension pneumothorax *(page 21)*.
- Cardiac arrest *(page 6)*.

possible signs, symptoms and treatment ? +

See 'Heart Conditions' (pages 24 - 25).

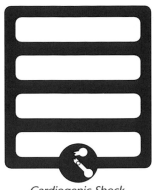

Cardiogenic Shock.

anaphylactic shock

Anaphylaxis is an extremely dangerous allergic reaction caused by a massive over-reaction of the body's immune system *(see page 18)*.

An anaphylactic reaction can cause shock because the large quantity of histamine released in the body makes:

- Blood vessels dilate *(causing a fall in blood pressure)*.
- Blood capillary walls become 'leaky' *(causing a fall in blood volume)*.
- The strength of the heart's contractions weaker *(causing a fall in blood pressure)*.

possible signs, symptoms and treatment ? +

See 'Anaphylaxis' (page 18)

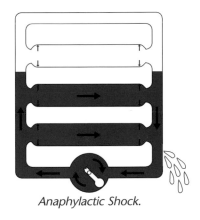

Anaphylactic Shock.

fainting

Fainting is caused by poor nervous control of the blood vessels and heart.

When a casualty faints, the blood vessels in the lower body dilate and the heart becomes slow. This results in the blood pressure falling and the patient has a temporary reduction in blood supply to the brain.

Typical causes of fainting are:

- Pain or fright.
- Lack of food.
- Emotional stress.

- Long periods of inactivity *(such as standing or sitting)*.
- Heat exhaustion *(page 43)*.

possible signs and symptoms ?

- Temporary loss of consciousness, falling to the floor.
- Slow pulse.
- Pale, clammy skin.

- Before the faint the casualty may have suffered nausea, stomach ache, blurred vision or dizziness.
- Quick recovery.

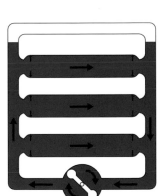

Fainting:
The heart slows and blood vessels dilate.

treatment of fainting +

- Lay the casualty down and raise their legs in the air, returning blood to the vital organs.
- Check **Airway** and **Breathing** *(page 6)*.
- Remove causes of stress, crowds of people and allow plenty of fresh air.
- Reassure the casualty as they recover. Do not allow them to sit up suddenly.
- If they feel faint again, repeat the treatment. Look for an underlying cause.
- If the casualty does not recover quickly or you are unsure: check airway and breathing again *(page 6)*, place them in the recovery position *(page 11)* and **dial 999 for an ambulance**.

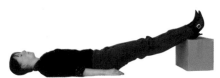

Fainting – lay the casualty down and raise the legs in the air.

circulation problems

hygiene when dealing with wounds

- Protect yourself by covering your own cuts and abrasions with a waterproof dressing, especially on your arms and hands.

- Wear disposable protective gloves and an apron when you are giving first aid.

- Use specialised cleaning agents for cleaning up body fluid spillages. Follow the instructions on the container and use disposable towels.

- Dispose of soiled dressings in a yellow 'clinical waste' bag. Destroy by incineration (send the bag to hospital with the casualty if you have no clinical waste facilities).

- Wash your hands thoroughly before and after dealing with a patient.

- If you regularly deal with body fluids, ask your doctor about vaccinations against Hepatitis 'B'.

wounds and bleeding

A wound can be defined as an abnormal break in the continuity of the tissues of the body. Any wound will to some extent result in bleeding, either internally or externally. If blood loss is severe, this could result in shock *(page 26)*, so urgent treatment would be necessary. This chapter deals with the different types of wound, the complications that may occur and their treatment.

types of wound and basic treatment

Contusion

A bruise. Caused by ruptured capillaries bleeding under the skin. This may have been the cause of a blunt blow, or by bleeding from underlying damage, such as a fracture.

- Cool the area with an ice pack or running water as soon as possible.

Abrasion

A graze. The top layers of skin are scraped off, usually as the result of a friction burn or sliding fall. Often containing particles of dirt, which could cause infection.

- Dirt that is not embedded should be removed using clean water and sterile swabs.

- Clean from the centre of the wound outwards, so as not to introduce more dirt into the wound.

Laceration

A rip or tear of the skin. More likely to have particles of dirt than a clean cut, although usually bleeds less.

- Treat for bleeding *(page 30)* and prevent infection.

Incision

A clean cut. Usually caused by a sharp object such as a knife. Deep wounds may involve complications such as severed tendons or blood vessels. This type of wound could 'gape open' and bleed profusely.

- Treat for bleeding *(page 30)* and prevent infection.

Puncture

A stabbing wound. Could be as a result of standing on a nail or being stabbed. The wound could be very deep and yet appear very small in diameter. Damage may be caused to underlying organs such as the heart or lungs and severe internal bleeding may occur.

- **Dial 999 for an ambulance** if you suspect damage to underlying organs or internal bleeding.

- Never remove an embedded object – it may be stemming bleeding and further damage may result.

Gun Shot

Caused by a bullet or other missile, which may be travelling at such speed as to drive into and then exit the body. A small entry wound could be accompanied by a large 'crater' exit wound. Severe bleeding and damage to organs usually results.

- **Dial 999 for Police and Ambulance.**

- Treat **Airway** and **Breathing** problems first *(pages 6 to 8)*.

- Pack the wound with dressings and try to prevent bleeding.

Amputation

Complete or partial severing of a limb.

- See treatment of amputation *(page 31)*.

De-gloved

Severing of the skin from the body, resulting in 'creasing' or a flap of skin, leaving a bare area of tissue. Caused by the force of the injuring object sliding along the length of the skin.

- Put the skin back in place if possible.

- Arrange urgent transport to hospital.

blood loss

How much blood do we have?

The amount of blood in our body varies in relation to our size. A rough rule of thumb is that we have approximately one pint of blood per stone in body weight, so the average adult has between 8 and 12 pints *(4.5 to 6.5 litres)* of blood, dependent on their size *(but the rule doesn't work for someone who is overweight)*.

Remember that children have less blood than adults, and as such can not afford to loose the same amount – a baby only has around **1 pint** of blood, so can only loose 1/3 of a pint before the blood pressure falls *(see below)*.

types of bleeding

Arterial Blood in the arteries is under direct pressure from the heart pumping and spurts in time with the heart beat. A wound to a major artery could result in blood '**spurting**' several metres and the blood volume will rapidly reduce. Blood in the arteries is rich in oxygen and is said to be 'bright red', however this can be difficult to assess. The most important factor is *how* the wound bleeds.

Venous Veins are not under direct pressure from the heart, but veins carry the same volume of blood as the arteries. A wound to a major vein may '**ooze**' profusely.

Capillary Bleeding from capillaries occurs in all wounds. Although the flow may appear fast at first, blood loss is usually slight and is easily controlled. Bleeding from a capillary could be described as a '**trickle**' of blood.

effects of blood loss ?

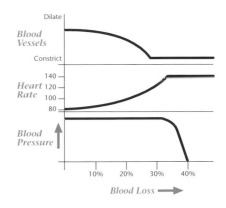

The table below show the effects, signs and symptoms of blood loss. Volumes of blood lost are given as a percentage, because we all have different amounts of blood.

As you can see, a loss of **30%** of blood volume is critical – the patient's condition rapidly deteriorates from this point onwards. Blood vessels cannot constrict any further and the heart cannot beat any faster, so blood pressure falls, resulting in unconsciousness and then death.

- Any patient with blood loss over 10% should be treated for shock *(page 26)*.

See also: *Hypovolaemic shock (page 26)*
          Hypoxia (page 14).

	10% Blood Loss	**20% Blood Loss**	**30% Blood Loss**	**40%+ Blood Loss**
Consciousness	Normal	May feel dizzy stood up	Lowered levels of consciousness. Restless, anxious	Unresponsive
Skin	Normal	Pale	Cyanosis *(blue grey tinges to the lips and skin)*, cold and clammy	Severe cyanosis, cold and clammy
Pulse	Normal *(this is the amount normally donated)*	Slightly raised	Rapid *(over 100 per min)* hard to detect	Undetectable
Breathing	Normal	Slightly raised	Rapid	Deep sighing breaths *(air hunger)*

wounds and bleeding

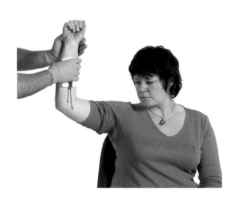

treatment of external bleeding

The aims of treatment for external bleeding are firstly to stop the bleeding, preventing the casualty from going into shock *(page 26),* and then to prevent infection.

S.E.E.P. will help you to remember the steps of treatment:

Sit or lay   Sit or lay the casualty down. Place them in a position that is appropriate to the location of the wound and the extent of their bleeding.

Examine   Examine the wound. Look for foreign objects and note how the wound is bleeding. Remember what it looks like, so you can describe it to medical staff when it's covered with a bandage.

Elevate   Elevate the wound. Ensure that the wound is above the level of the heart, using gravity to reduce the blood flow to the injury.

Pressure   Apply **direct** or **indirect** pressure to stem bleeding:

direct pressure

The best way to stem bleeding is by applying direct pressure over the wound. Immediate pressure can temporarily be applied with the hands, however you should take precautions to prevent yourself from coming into contact with the patient's blood, preferably by wearing disposable gloves. The pressure should be continuous for 10 minutes. A firm bandage *(not so tight as to stop circulation to the limb altogether!)* is usually sufficient to stop bleeding from most minor wounds. If there is an embedded object in the wound, you may be able to apply pressure at either side of the object.

indirect pressure

If direct pressure for a wound on a limb is not possible or effective, indirect pressure can be used as a last resort. Pressure can be applied to the artery supplying the limb, squashing it against a bone and reducing the blood flow. Apply indirect pressure for a maximum of 10 minutes.

The two main indirect pressure points are:

Brachial   Pressure is applied to the brachial artery, which runs on the inside of the upper arm. One way of doing this is to get the patient to make a fist with their opposite hand, place it under their arm pit and squeeze the injured arm down onto the fist.

Femoral   Pressure is applied to the femoral artery, which is located where the thigh bone *(femur)* crosses the 'bikini line'. Take care to explain your actions. One way of doing this is to use the heel of your foot to apply the pressure.

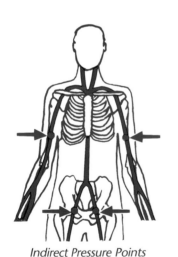

Indirect Pressure Points

dressings

A dressing should be sterile and just large enough to cover the wound. It should be absorbent and preferably made of material that won't stick to the clotting blood *(a 'non-adherent' dressing).*

A firmly applied dressing is sufficient to stem bleeding from the majority of minor wounds, but the dressing should not restrict blood flow to the rest of the limb *(check the circulation with a 'capillary refill' test, page 23)*

Extra pressure 'by hand' and elevation may be necessary for severe bleeding. If the dressing becomes saturated with blood, keep it in place and put another larger dressing on top. If this doesn't work take the dressings off and start again.

Embedded objects in a wound should not be removed. Use sterile dressings and bandages to 'build up' around the protruding object. This will apply pressure around the wound and support the object. Arrange for the casualty to go to hospital to have the object removed.

NEVER try to stop bleeding by tying a band around the limb (a tourniquet) – it may cause tissue damage or make the bleeding worse.

NEVER remove an embedded object – it may be stemming bleeding and further damage may result.

amputation

Amputation is the complete or partial severing of a limb, and is extremely traumatic for the patient. Modern microsurgery techniques now make the re-plantation of amputated limbs possible, however the majority of amputated body parts are still lost, so you should not make blind promises to a patient.

- Treat the casualty for bleeding *(page 30)* and for shock *(page 26)*. Indirect pressure may be necessary to control the bleeding.
- **Dial 999 for an ambulance.**
- Dress the casualty's wound with a non-adherent, non-fluffy dressing.
- Wrap the amputated limb in a plastic bag, and then place the package onto a pack of ice to preserve it. Do not allow the limb to come into direct contact with the ice or water.

NEVER place an amputated limb directly into ice or water. The limb should be wrapped in a plastic bag to keep it dry.

internal bleeding

Internal bleeding is a very serious condition, yet can be very difficult to recognise in its early stages. Internal bleeding can be as a result of injury, such as lung or abdominal injuries, yet can also happen 'spontaneously' to an apparently well patient, such as bleeding from a stomach ulcer or a weak artery.

Although blood may not actually be lost 'externally' from the body, it is lost out of the arteries and veins, so shock can quickly develop.

Other serious life threatening complications can occur from internal bleeding, such as a brain haemorrhage or bleeding into the lungs.

possible signs and symptoms

You should suspect internal bleeding if signs of shock *(see pages 26 and 29)* are present, but there is no obvious cause, such as external bleeding.

There may be:

- Signs of SHOCK *(page 26)*.
- Pain, or a history of recent pain at the site of bleeding.
- Bruising and/or swelling.
- Other symptoms related to the site of bleeding *(e.g. difficulty breathing if the bleeding is in the lung)*.

Internal bleeding in certain areas of the body may result in an external show of blood. The blood may be mixed with the contents of the organ from where it originated:

Bleeding from	Appearance	Possible causes
Ear	Bright red or clots	Perforated ear drum, fractured skull
	Blood with a 'watered down' appearance	Fractured skull, leaking cerebrospinal fluid from around the brain
Nose	Bright red or clots	Nose bleed
	Blood with a 'watered down' appearance	Fractured skull, leaking cerebrospinal fluid from around the brain
Mouth	Bright red, frothy	Bleeding in the lungs
	Vomited, or brown 'coffee grounds' appearance	Bleeding in the stomach
Urethra	Smoky red colour	Bleeding in the kidneys or bladder
Vagina	Fresh blood or clots	Menstruation, miscarriage, injury or disease to the vagina or womb
Anus	Bright red fresh blood	Bleeding from the lower bowel/rectum. Possibly haemorrhoids or injury
	Black 'offensive smelling' stools	Bleeding from the large intestines/bowel

treatment of internal bleeding

- *Dial 999 for an ambulance.*
- *Treat the casualty for shock as necessary (page 26).*

wounds and bleeding

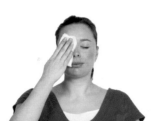

Make sure the patient keeps the good eye closed.

eye injury

Small particles of dust or dirt can be washed out of the patient's eye with cold tap water. Ensure the water runs away from the good eye.

For a more serious eye injury:

- Keep the patient still and give them a soft sterile dressing to gently hold over the injured eye. This can be carefully bandaged in place later if necessary.

- Tell the casualty to close their good eye, because any movement of this will cause the injured eye to move also. If necessary, bandage the good eye to stop the patient using it. Lots of reassurance will be needed!

- Take the casualty to hospital. **Dial 999 for an ambulance** if necessary.

For chemicals in the eye:

- Wash with copious amounts of clean water, ensuring water runs away from the good eye. **Dial 999 for an ambulance** *(also see 'chemical burns', page 33).*

nose bleeds

Weakened or dried out blood vessels in the nose can rupture as a result of a bang to the nose, picking or blowing it. More serious causes could be high blood pressure or a fractured skull.

- Sit the patient down, head tipped forward.

- Nip the soft part of the nose. Maintain constant pressure for 10 minutes.

- Tell the patient to breathe through the mouth.

- Give the patient a cloth to mop up any blood whilst the nose is nipped.

- Advise the patient not to breathe through or blow their nose for a few hours after bleeding has stopped.

- If bleeding persists for more than 30 minutes, or if the patient takes 'anticoagulant' drugs *(such as warfarin)*, take or send them to hospital in an upright position.

- Advise a patient suffering from frequent nosebleeds to visit their doctor.

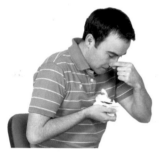

Nip the soft part of the nose. Maintain constant pressure for 10 minutes.

crush injury

Crush injuries most commonly occur as a result of building site or traffic accidents. If the blood flow to a limb *(e.g. an arm or a leg)* is impaired by the weight of a crushing object, there is a danger of toxins building up in the muscle tissues below the site of the crushing.

If the blood flow to the limb is impaired for 15 minutes or more, the toxins will build up so much that if they are released into the rest of the body *(which will happen when the crushing object is removed)* they may cause kidney failure. This is called 'crush syndrome' and may result in death.

Expert medical care is needed when releasing the patient if the blood flow has been impaired for 15 minutes or more.

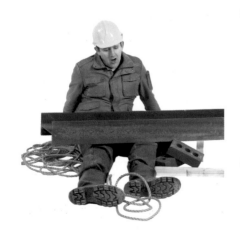

treatment for crushing less than 15 minutes

- Release the casualty as quickly as possible if you can.
- **Dial 999 for an ambulance.**
- Control any bleeding and cover open wounds.
- Treat for shock if necessary *(page 26)*, taking care not to move injuries.
- Monitor **Airway** and **Breathing** until help arrives.

treatment for crushing more than 15 minutes

- DO NOT release the casualty.
- **Dial 999 for an ambulance.** Give clear information about the incident.
- Monitor **Airway** and **Breathing** until help arrives.

causes of burns and treatment

The different causes of burn can be separated in to 5 areas. The treatment for the burn can differ slightly depending on the cause:

dry heat burns

Any direct contact with a dry heat source or friction.

- Do not put yourself in danger.

- Ensure that **Airway** and **Breathing** are maintained *(page 6)*.

- **Cool** the burn immediately with cold *(preferably running)* water, for at least 10 minutes. If water is not available, any cold harmless liquid *(milk, pop etc.)* is better than no cooling at all. Do this first then move quickly to a water supply if you can. Take care not to cool large areas of burns so much that you induce hypothermia.

- **Remove** watches, rings etc. during cooling, as burned areas will swell. Clothing that has not stuck to the wound may be removed carefully.

- **Dress** the wound with a sterile non-adherent dressing. Cling film is one of the best dressings for a burn – the inside of the roll should be sterile, and it will not stick to the burn. Ensure the wound has been cooled beforehand. Do not wrap cling film around a limb – lay it over the burn. Alternatives could be a clean plastic bag, or specialised burns dressings.

- See note *(overleaf)* on when to refer a burns patient to hospital.

- **Dial 999 for an ambulance** if the burn appears severe, or the casualty has breathed in smoke or fumes.

wet heat (scalds)

Scalds are most commonly from hot water, but may be from hot fats or other liquids that can reach higher temperatures than water.

- Treat as a dry heat burn.

chemical burns

Caused by chemicals which either corrode the skin or create heat *(or both)*.

- Make the area safe – contain the chemical, and protect yourself from coming into contact with it.

- Irrigate the burn with lots of running water to wash the chemical away. This should be done for longer than a thermal burn – at least 20 minutes.

- **Dial 999 for an ambulance.** Make a note of the chemical, and give this information to the ambulance operator if possible.

- Remove contaminated clothing carefully whilst irrigating the burn.

- If an eye is contaminated, irrigate as above, but ensure that the water runs away from the un-affected eye.

- Some chemicals in the workplace cannot be safely diluted with water – health and safety regulations require an 'antidote' to be available in an emergency. You should be trained in the use of the antidote.

radiation burns (sun burn)

Most commonly seen as sunburn.

- Remove the casualty from exposure of the sun and cool the area with cold water for 10 minutes.

- If there is extensive blistering, or you are not sure, seek medical advice.

- Give the casualty frequent sips of water to ensure that heat exhaustion does not take effect *(page 43)*.

- If the sunburn is mild, after-sun cream or calamine lotion may soothe the area.

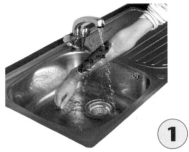

Cool the burn for 10 minutes.

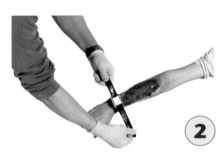

Remove jewellery and LOOSE clothing.

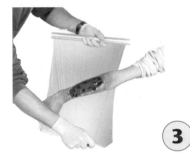

Dress the burn. Cling film is one of the best dressings for a burn.

NEVER burst blisters (the layer of skin is protecting against infection)

NEVER touch the burn.

NEVER apply lotions, ointments or fats – they might introduce infection, and would need to be removed in hospital.

NEVER apply adhesive tape or dressings – the burn may be larger than it first appears.

NEVER remove clothing that has stuck to the burn.

electric burns

Caused by heat that is generated by an electrical current flowing through the tissues of the body. You may be able to see a burn where the current entered the body, and at the point of exit. There may be deep internal burns which are not visible along the path of the current flow. The extent of the internal burns can be estimated by the severity of the entry and exit wounds.

An electric shock may cause cardiac arrest. In this case, **Airway** and **Breathing** become the priority.

- Ensure your own safety – make sure contact with the electricity is broken.

- Ensure **Airway** and **Breathing** are maintained *(pages 6 to 8)*.

- Irrigate the area of the burns, including the path between entry and exit, for at least 10 minutes.

- **Dial 999 for an ambulance.**

- Continue treatment as you would for a 'dry heat' burn.

estimating the severity of a burn

There are 5 factors that combine to affect the severity of a burn:

Size — The larger the area of the burn, the more severe. The size of the burn is given as a percentage of the body's surface area. An easy way to work this out is to compare the size of the burn with the patient's hand. An area equal to the size of the palm of the patient's opened hand *(including fingers)* is equal to **1%** of their body area.

Cause — The cause of the burn, as previously described in this chapter, will influence the overall severity – for example, electrical burns may leave a patient with deep internal burns. Some chemicals *(such as hydrofluoric acid)* could cause poisoning in addition to burns.

Age — The age of the patient will affect the recovery rate and severity. Babies and young children will burn at lower temperatures than adults. Elderly patient's burns take longer to heal and they may be more susceptible to infection.

Location — The location of the burn can affect the severity – in particular burns to the airway of a patient by inhaling hot gasses can be an instant killer. Burns to the eye may result in blindness.

Depth — The deeper the burn, the more severe. *See depth of burns below.*

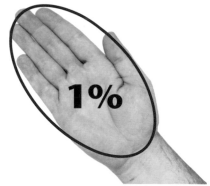

An area equal to the size of the palm of the patient's opened hand (including fingers) is equal to 1% of their body area.

Refer a burns patient to hospital if:

- *The burn is larger than 1-inch square.*

- *The patient is a child.*

- *The burn goes all the way around a limb.*

- *Any part of the burn appears to be full thickness.*

- *The burn involves hands, feet, genitals or the face.*

- *You are not sure.*

depth of burns

The skin consists of 3 layers – the 'epidermis' on the outside, the 'dermis' beneath, which lies on a layer of 'subcutaneous' fat.

The depth of burns can be defined as:

Superficial — This involves only the outer epidermis layer, and most commonly occurs from scalds. The burn looks red, sore and swollen.

Intermediate — This affects both the epidermis and the dermis layers of skin. The burn looks raw and blisters will form.

Full Thickness — The layers of skin are burned away to the subcutaneous fat layer or beyond. The burn may look pale, charred or waxy. The nerve endings will be burned away, so pain in this area may be absent, misleading both you and the patient.

the skeletal system

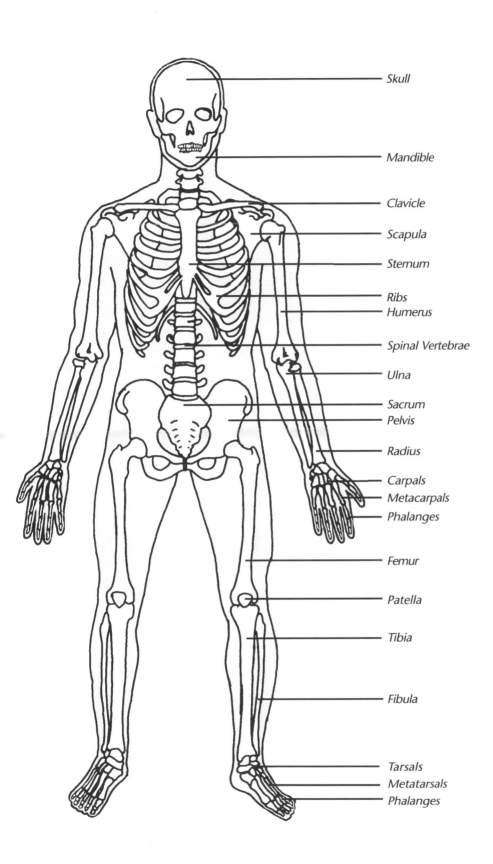

Skull

Mandible

Clavicle

Scapula

Sternum

Ribs
Humerus

Spinal Vertebrae

Ulna

Sacrum
Pelvis

Radius

Carpals
Metacarpals
Phalanges

Femur

Patella

Tibia

Fibula

Tarsals
Metatarsals
Phalanges

The skeleton consists of 206 bones, the functions of which are to:

- Provide support for the soft tissues of the body. This gives the body its shape.

- Provide protection for important organs such as the brain, lungs and spinal cord.

- Allow movement, by incorporating different types of joints and attachment for muscles.

- Produce red blood cells, some white blood cells and platelets in the marrow of bones such as the femur.

- Provide a store of minerals and energy such as calcium and fats.

injuries to bone, muscles and joints

causes of injury

Injury can be caused to the bones, muscles and joints by different types of force:

Direct Force   Damage results at the location where the force was applied, e.g. as the result of a blow or kick.

Indirect Force   Damage occurs away from the point where the force was applied, e.g. a fractured collar bone, as a result of landing on an outstretched arm.

Twisting Force   Damage results from torsion forces on the bones and muscles, Force e.g. 'twisting an ankle'.

Violent Movement   Injury results from a sudden violent movement, such as injuring the knee joint by kicking violently.

Pathological   Injury results because the bones have become brittle or weak, due to disease or old age.

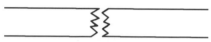

Closed Fracture

types of fracture

A fracture can be defined as a 'break in the continuity of the bone'. The basic categories of fracture are:

Closed   This is a clean break or crack in the bone, with no complications.

Open   The skin has become broken by the bone which may *(or may not)* still be protruding from the wound. This type of injury has a high risk of infection.

Complicated   With this type of injury, there are complications which have arisen as a result of the fracture, such as trapped blood vessels or nerves.

Green Stick   This type of fracture occurs more commonly in children, who have young, more flexible bone. The bone is split, but not totally severed. Green Stick fractures are often mistaken for sprains and strains, because only a few of the signs and symptoms of a fracture are present.

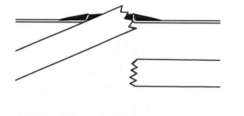

Open Fracture

dislocations

A dislocation is where a bone becomes partially or fully dislodged at a joint, usually as a result of wrenching movement or sudden muscular contraction. The most common dislocations are the knee cap, shoulder, jaw, thumb or a finger.

There may also be a fracture at or near the site of the dislocation, and damage to ligaments, tendons and cartilage. It can be difficult to distinguish between a fracture and a dislocation.

Never attempt to manipulate a dislocated joint back into place. This is a job for the experts – the procedure can be extremely painful for the patient, and you may cause further damage.

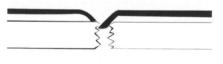

Complicated Fracture

sprains and strains

A *sprain* is defined as an injury to a ligament at a joint. A *strain* is defined as an injury to muscle. Usually caused by sudden wrenching movements, the joint overstretches, tearing the surrounding muscle or ligament.

Minor fractures are commonly mistaken for sprains and strains. If you are not sure, you should treat the injury as if it was a fracture. The only way to rule out a fracture is by x-ray.

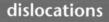

Green Stick Fracture

for treatment of sprains and strains – see page 38

possible signs and symptoms of a fracture ?

The following mnemonic can be used to help you remember the signs and symptoms of a fracture:

Pain
At the site of the fracture. Strong pain killers, nerve damage or dementia may mask the pain, so beware.

Loss of Power
e.g. not being able to lift anything with a fractured arm.

Unnatural movement
This type of fracture is classed as 'unstable' and care should be taken to prevent the fracture from moving.

Swelling or bruising
Around the site of the fracture.

Deformity
If a leg is bent in the wrong place, it's broken!

Irregularity
Lumps or depressions along the surface of the bone, where the broken ends of the bone overlap.

Crepitus
The feeling and sound of bone grating on bone, when the broken ends rub on each other.

Tenderness
At the site of the injury.

treatment of a basic fracture ✚

See also:
Head Injuries *(pages 12 to 13)*

Flail Chest *(page 21)*

Spinal Injuries *(pages 38 to 39)*

- Reassure the casualty, tell them to keep still.
- Keep injury still with your hands until it is properly immobilised. The casualty might be able to do this on their own.
- Don't move the casualty until the injury is immobilised, unless they are in danger.
- Don't try to bandage an injury if you have called an ambulance, just keep it still *(cover open wounds with a sterile dressing)*.
- Don't let the casualty eat or drink – they may need an operation.

for an upper limb injury:

- Carefully place the arm in a sling against the trunk of the body. Arm fractures are normally placed in a support sling. Collar bone fractures are normally supported by an elevated sling *(keep the elbow down at the patient's side when using an elevated sling for a collar bone fracture)*.
- If the casualty is in severe pain, circulation or nerves to the arm are affected, the casualty has breathing difficulties, or you are unsure, **dial 999 for an ambulance.**
- Arrange transport to hospital.

for a lower limb injury:

- Keep the casualty warm and still. **Dial 999 for an ambulance.**
- If the ambulance arrival will be delayed *(e.g. remote countryside)* immobilise the injury by bandaging the sound leg to the injured one.
- Check circulation beyond the injury and any bandages. Loosen bandages if necessary.

support sling

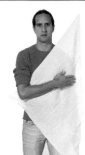

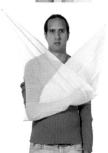

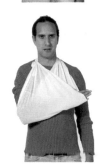

elevated sling

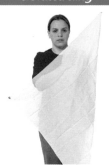

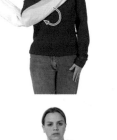

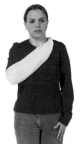

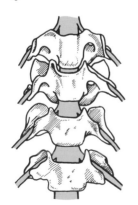

treatment of sprains and strains

The best treatment for a sprain or strain is to follow the RICE mnemonic:

Rest — Rest the injury. e.g. don't allow a sports player to carry on playing *(it's better to take time out now than miss the next ten matches!)*.

Ice — Apply an ice pack to the injury as soon as possible. This will help reduce swelling, which will speed recovery. Place a tea towel or triangular bandage between the skin and the ice pack. Do this for 10 minutes, every 2 hours, for 24 hours for maximum effect.

Compression — Apply a firm *(not constrictive)* bandage to the injured area. This helps to reduce swelling. The bandage can be applied over a crushed ice pack for the first 10 minutes.

Elevation — Elevate the injury. This also reduces swelling.

Remember: minor fractures can easily be mistaken for sprains and strains. The only way to rule out a fracture is by x-ray, so take or send the casualty to hospital.

CAUTION: *To prevent frostbite always wrap the ice pack in a cloth and apply it for a maximum of 10 minutes. Allow the skin to return to normal temperature before repeat applications.*

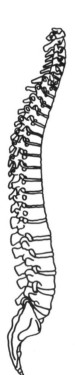

7 Cervical Vertebrae

12 Thoracic Vertebrae

5 Lumbar Vertebrae

5 Fused Sacral Vertebrae

spinal injuries

Spinal injury occurs with approximately 2% of trauma *(injury)* patients. Although this figure appears relatively low, suspecting and correctly treating the injury is essential, because poor treatment of a patient with a spinal injury could result in them becoming crippled for life or even death.

The spinal cord is an extension of the brain stem, and travels down the back of the spinal vertebrae. Vital nerves, controlling breathing and movement of limbs travel down the spinal cord *(see diagram)*. The weakest part of the spinal column is the neck, and indeed a neck injury can be the most severe type of spinal injury, because the nerves controlling breathing may become severed.

suspect spinal injury if the casualty has:

- Sustained a blow to the head, neck or back *(especially resulting in unconsciousness)*.
- Fallen from a height *(e.g. fall from a horse)*.
- Dived into shallow water.
- Been in an accident involving speed *(e.g. car accident or knocked down)*.
- Been involved in a 'cave in' accident *(e.g. crushing, or collapsed rugby scrum)*.
- Multiple injuries.
- Pain or tenderness in the neck or back after an accident *(pain killers or other severe injuries may mask the pain – beware)*.
- OR: if you are in any doubt.

The spinal cord travels through the centre of the spinal column. Nerves emanate from each vertebrae in pairs.

possible signs and symptoms of spinal injury

Remember – If some of these signs and symptoms are present, nerves may already be damaged. You should treat a patient who you _suspect_ has an injury to _prevent_ these signs and symptoms from developing.

- Pain or tenderness in the neck or back.
- Signs of a fracture in the neck or back *(page 37)*.
- Loss of control of limbs at or below the site of injury.
- Loss of feeling in the limbs.
- Sensations in the limbs, such as pins and needles or burning.
- Breathing difficulties.
- Incontinence.

treatment of spinal injury

if the patient is conscious:

- Reassure the patient. Tell them not to move.
- Keep the patient in the position you find them. Do not allow them to move, unless they are in severe danger.
- Hold their head still with your hands. Keep the head and neck in line with the upper body *(see diagram)*.
- **Dial 999 for an ambulance.** Keep the patient still and warm until it arrives.

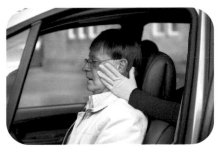

Holding a patient's head still in a car.

if the patient is unconscious and breathing normally:

- Do not move the patient unless they are in severe danger.
- If the patient is breathing normally this means the airway must be clear, so there is no need to tip the head back. The 'jaw thrust' technique can be used to keep the airway open without moving the head *(this is explained on page 40)*. Constantly monitor breathing.
- **Dial 999 for an ambulance.**
- Hold the head still with your hands. Keep the head and neck in line with the upper body *(see diagram)*.
- If you have to **leave** the casualty, if they begin to **vomit**, or if you are concerned about their **airway** in any way, place the casualty in the **recovery position**. Keep the head, neck and upper body in line as you turn the patient. Doing this effectively takes more than one rescuer, so get local help if you can *(see page 40 for methods of turning a spinal injury patient)*.
- Keep the casualty warm and still. Constantly monitor **Airway** and **Breathing** until help arrives *(page 6)*.

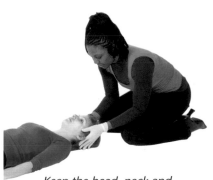

Keep the head, neck and upper body in line.

if the patient is not breathing normally:

- If the patient is not breathing normally, the airway will need to be opened. Head tilt may be used, but the tilt should be the minimum that is required to allow unobstructed rescue breaths.
- **Only** if you are trained and confident, you can try the 'jaw thrust' technique to open the airway, but if you find the patient is still not breathing normally, you should then open the airway using the head tilt method before carrying out resuscitation *(page 6)*.
- Re-check breathing once the airway has been opened.
- If the casualty is still not breathing normally, **dial 999 for an ambulance,** then carry out resuscitation *(pages 6 to 8)*.
- Obtain the help of others to support the head as you resuscitate.

Remember – successful resuscitation that results in paralysis from a neck injury is a tragedy, but failing to maintain an adequate airway will result in death.

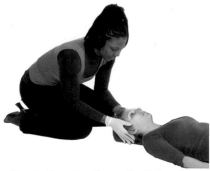

Fig. 1: Keeping the patient's head and neck in line with the body.

managing the airway with spinal injuries

If a patient is unconscious and laid on their back, the airway can be in danger from vomit or the tongue falling back.

A patient who has not been injured can simply be turned into the recovery position to protect the airway, but if spinal injuries are suspected, great care must be taken not to move the spine.

If a patient is already on their side *(not on their back)* you may not have to move them at all. Is the airway in danger from vomit or the tongue falling back? If not, the patient can be kept still in the position you find them.

If you can continually monitor that the patient is breathing normally, you may be able to keep them still until the ambulance arrives, even if they are on their back.

If the tongue begins to fall back or the patient vomits however, immediate action will be needed to protect the airway.

jaw thrust

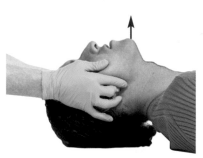

Fig. 2: The jaw thrust technique. Use your middle and index fingers to lift the jaw whilst you keep the head still.

If the patient is breathing but the tongue is starting to obstruct the airway *(usually makes snoring type noises)* the jaw thrust technique can be used to keep the airway open:

- Kneel above the head of the patient, knees apart to give you balance.
- With your elbows resting on your legs *(or the floor)* for support, hold the patient's head with your hands to keep their head and neck in line with the body *(see fig.1)*.
- Place the middle and index fingers of your hands under the jaw line of the patient *(under their ears)*.
- Keeping the head still, lift the jaw upwards with your fingers *(see fig.2)*. This gently lifts the tongue from the back of the throat.

DO NOT *attampt the jaw thrust technique during CPR - tilt the head to open the airway instead (page 6).*

log roll

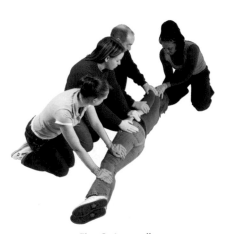

Fig. 3: Log roll.

If you have to **leave** the casualty, if they begin to **vomit**, or if you are concerned about their **airway** in any way, the patient will have to be turned onto their side. The head, neck and upper body must be kept in line as you turn the patient.

The best method of turning a spinal injury patient is the log roll technique, but you will need at least three helpers to roll the patient.

- Support the head of the patient, keeping the head, neck and upper body in line *(see fig.1)*.
- Your helpers should kneel along one side of the patient. Get them to gently straighten the patient's legs and arms.
- Making sure that everyone works together, the helpers should roll the patient towards them on your count. You gently move the head to follow the body as the patient is rolled. *(see fig.3)*.
- Keep the head, neck, body and legs in line at all times. If you can, keep the patient in this position until the ambulance arrives.

recovery position

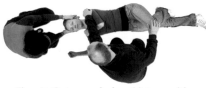

Fig. 4: Get your helper(s) to position the patient's arm and legs ready for the recovery position.

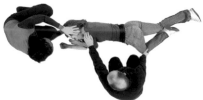

Fig. 5: Get your helper(s) to turn the patient whilst you keep the head in line with the body.

If the patient has to be turned onto their side and you don't have three helpers, you will need to use the recovery position method when turning the patient. Keep the head, neck and body in line as best as you can as you roll the patient over. Have some padding *(e.g. a folded coat)* to support the patient's head when they are on their side.

If you have one or two helpers, you can support the head as your helper(s) turn the patient.

- Start by supporting the head of the patient, keeping the head, neck and upper body in line *(see fig.1)*.
- Get your helper(s) to gently move the patient's arms and legs into position, ready to turn the patient into the recovery position *(see fig.4)*.
- Making sure that everyone works together, the helper(s) should roll the patient into the recovery position. The helper(s) should pull equally on the patient's far leg and shoulder as they turn the patient, keeping the spine in line. You gently move the head to keep it in line with the body as the patient is moved *(see fig.5)*.

body temperature

The body works best when its temperature is close to 37°C *(98.6°F)*. This temperature is maintained by an area in the centre of the brain called the *'hypothalamus'*.

If the body becomes too hot we produce sweat, which evaporates and cools the skin. Blood vessels near to the skin dilate *(flushed skin)* and the cooled blood is circulated around the body.

If the body becomes too cold we shiver, which creates heat by muscle movement. Blood vessels near to the skin constrict *(pale skin)*, keeping the blood close to the warmer core of the body. Hairs on the skin become erect, trapping warm air *(goose pimples)*.

Injuries resulting from exposure to extremes of temperature can be 'localised' *(such as sunburn or frostbite)*, or 'generalised' *(such as hypothermia or heat stroke)*.

signs and symptoms of body temperature change ?

The symptoms of over-exposure to heat or cold are demonstrated by the diagram below. As the temperature of the body becomes too hot or too cold, the area of the brain that regulates temperature *(the hypothalamus)* stops working, and the condition rapidly becomes worse as the body no longer fights the condition:

This chapter covers the effects of over exposure to heat or cold on the body.

Severe Hypothermia or Heat Stroke are potentially fatal conditions, and need skillful treatment from the First Aider.

The people who are most at risk from the effects of heat and cold are the elderly or infirm, babies and children, or people who take part in outdoor activities such as hiking or sailing.

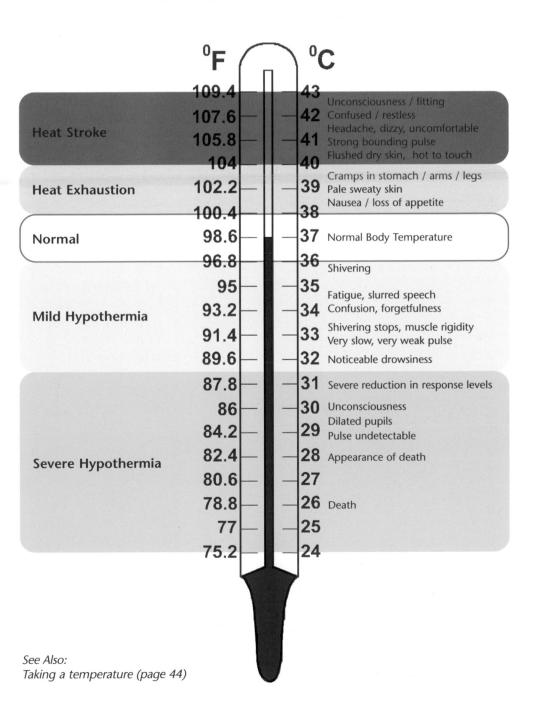

	°F	°C	
Heat Stroke	109.4	43	Unconsciousness / fitting
	107.6	42	Confused / restless
	105.8	41	Headache, dizzy, uncomfortable / Strong bounding pulse
	104	40	Flushed dry skin, hot to touch
Heat Exhaustion	102.2	39	Cramps in stomach / arms / legs / Pale sweaty skin
	100.4	38	Nausea / loss of appetite
Normal	98.6	37	Normal Body Temperature
	96.8	36	Shivering
	95	35	
Mild Hypothermia	93.2	34	Fatigue, slurred speech / Confusion, forgetfulness
	91.4	33	Shivering stops, muscle rigidity / Very slow, very weak pulse
	89.6	32	Noticeable drowsiness
	87.8	31	Severe reduction in response levels
	86	30	Unconsciousness
	84.2	29	Dilated pupils / Pulse undetectable
Severe Hypothermia	82.4	28	Appearance of death
	80.6	27	
	78.8	26	Death
	77	25	
	75.2	24	

See Also:
Taking a temperature (page 44)

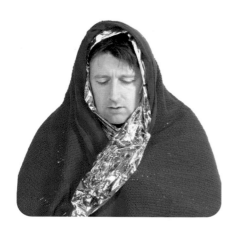

hypothermia

The onset of hypothermia occurs when the body's core temperature falls below 35°C. A patient suffering hypothermia in its mildest form who is treated effectively will usually make a full recovery. If the body's core temperature falls below 26°C the condition will most likely be fatal, however resuscitation has been successful on people with temperatures as low as 10°C, so it is always worth attempting.

The underlying cause of hypothermia is over exposure to cold temperatures, however different conditions and types of patient will increase the risk:

- The hypothalamus *(temperature control centre)* of a baby or young child is under developed, and hypothermia can result from as little as being in a cold room.

- Elderly or infirm patients do not generate as much body heat, so prolonged periods in a cold environment can lower the core temperature.

- Wet clothing, or immersion in cold water results in the body cooling much faster than it would in dry air. Water conducts heat away from the body.

- A person who is not clothed properly in windy conditions will have cold air continually in contact with the skin, resulting in faster cooling of the body.

possible signs and symptoms

- Pale skin, cold to touch.

- Shivering at first, then muscle stiffness as the body cools further.

- Slowing of the body's functions – including thought, speech, pulse and breathing *(the pulse can fall lower than 40 beats per minute)*.

- Lethargy, confusion, disorientation *(can be mistaken for drunkenness)*.

- Lowered levels of response, eventually unconsciousness, then death.

treatment

if the casualty is unconscious:

- Open the **Airway** and check **Breathing**. Resuscitate if necessary *(pages 6 to 8)*.

- **Dial 999 for an ambulance.**

- Gently place the patient in the recovery position *(page 11)*. Do not move the patient unnecessarily, because the slightest jolt can stop the heart.

- Place blankets or other insulating materials under and around the patient. Cover the head.

- Constantly monitor breathing. The pulse may be hard to find – it is safe to assume the heart is beating if the casualty is breathing normally.

for a conscious casualty:

- If you can shelter the casualty, remove any wet clothing. Quickly replace with dry, warm garments. Cover the head.

- If the casualty is fit, young and able to climb into a bath without help, bathe them in warm water *(40°C / 104°F)*. **Don't allow an elderly patient to bathe.**

- If a bath is not possible, wrap them in warm blankets. Heat the room to a warm temperature *(25°C / 77°F)* if indoors.

- A casualty outdoors should be insulated from the environment and ground. Use a survival bag and shelter if available. Share your body heat with them.

- Give the casualty warm drinks and food.

- **Seek medical advice** if the patient is elderly, a child, or if you are in any doubt about their condition.

- If the condition seems severe. **Dial 999 for an ambulance.**

NEVER give a patient alcohol (it dilates blood vessels, which will make the patient colder).

NEVER place direct sources of heat on or near the patient (they draw blood to the skin, causing a fall in blood pressure and place stress on the heart).

NEVER warm babies or the elderly too quickly (e.g. by placing them in a warm bath).

BEWARE: A hypothermic heart is in grave risk of 'ventricular fibrillation', which causes cardiac arrest. Handle hypothermic patients with care – the slightest jolt can induce the condition.

frostbite

Frostbite is a condition caused when an extremity *(such as a finger or an ear)* is subject to cold conditions. The cells of the limb become frozen. Ice crystals form in the cells, which causes them to rupture and die. Frostbite may also be accompanied by hypothermia, which should also be treated. Serious frostbite can result in the complete loss of a limb, particularly fingers or toes.

possible signs and symptoms ?

- Pins and needles, followed by numbness.
- Hardening and stiffening of the skin.
- Skin colour change – first white, then blue tinges, then eventually black.
- On recovery, the injury will become hot, red, blistered and very painful.

treatment

- **Gently** remove rings, watches etc.
- Stop the freezing becoming worse if the casualty is still outdoors – place the limb under their arm or hold it with your hands.
- Don't rub the injury – this will cause damage.
- Don't re-warm the injury if there is a risk of it refreezing. Move the patient indoors before you treat them.
- Place the injury in warm water *(test the temperature with your elbow as you would for a baby's bath – not with a frozen hand!)*.
- An adult casualty can take two paracetamol tablets for intense pain.
- Take the casualty to hospital as soon as possible.

heat exhaustion

Heat exhaustion is the body's response to loss of water and salt through excessive sweating. The most common cause of this condition is working or exercising in hot conditions *(such as hiking on a very hot day)*.

Heat exhaustion occurs when the core body temperature raises above 38°C. If the problem is not treated, it can quickly lead to heat stroke *(overleaf)*.

possible signs and symptoms ?

- Confusion, dizziness.
- Pale, sweaty skin.
- Nausea, loss of appetite, vomiting.
- Fast, weak pulse and breathing.
- Cramps in the arms, legs, abdomen.
- The casualty may say that they 'feel cold', but they will be hot to touch.

treatment

- Take the casualty to a cool place.
- Remove excessive clothing and lay them down.
- Give the casualty plenty of drinks of water to re-hydrate them. If possible, add one level teaspoon of salt per litre of water.
- Obtain medical advice, even if the casualty recovers quickly.
- If the casualty's levels of response *(page 9)* deteriorate – place them in the recovery position and **dial 999 for an ambulance.** Monitor **Airway** and **Breathing** *(page 6)*.
- Treat for heat stroke *(overleaf)* as necessary.

Trench Foot

This is caused by prolonged exposure to wet, cold conditions. The cells do not freeze, so full recovery is usual. The symptoms and treatment are similar to frostbite.

Chilblains

The most common cold injury, caused by exposure to dry cold. Again the cells do not freeze. There may be itching, reddish-blue skin and swelling. With time, blisters may form. Treat as frostbite.

NEVER rub the affected area.

NEVER use direct or dry heat to warm the injury.

NEVER re-warm the injury if there is a danger of it refreezing.

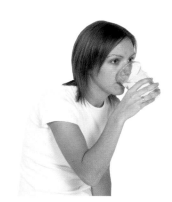

Give the casualty plenty of drinks of water to re-hydrate them.

effects of heat and cold

heat stroke

Heat stroke is a very serious condition. It results from failure of the hypothalamus *(temperature control centre)* in the brain. The sweating mechanism fails, the body is unable to cool down and the core temperature can reach dangerously high levels *(over 40°C)* within 10 to 15 minutes.

The condition can be caused by a high fever or prolonged exposure to heat and often follows heat exhaustion *(previous page).*

possible signs and symptoms

- Severe confusion and restlessness.
- Flushed, hot, dry skin *(no sweating).*
- Strong, fast pulse.
- Throbbing headache.
- Dizziness.
- Nausea, vomiting.
- Reduction in levels of response *(page 9)* leading to unconsciousness.
- Possibility of fitting if unconscious.

treatment

- Move the casualty to a cool, shaded area.
- **Dial 999 for an ambulance.**
- Cool the casualty rapidly, using whatever methods you can:
  - Remove outer clothing, and wrap the casualty in a cold, wet sheet. Keep it wet and cold until the casualty's temperature falls to normal levels.
- Other methods of cooling can be:
  - continually sponging with cold water, and fanning the casualty to help it evaporate.
  - placing in a cool shower if they are conscious enough to do so.
  - spraying with cool water from a garden hose.
- If the casualty fits, treat as you would for a febrile convulsion *(page 50).*

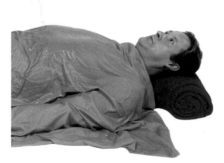

Cool the casualty rapidly.

'Recreational' Drugs

In recent years ambulance services have seen an increase in the use of so called 'recreational' drugs such as ecstasy (or 'e').

A casualty under the influence of such a drug may dance continually for long periods, which causes them to sweat excessively, and thus become hot and dehydrated.

The effects of dehydration, combined with the drug affecting 'normal' thought, can lead to heat exhaustion and heat stroke.

taking a temperature

Modern, easy to use thermometers are now available, such as disposable strips that can be placed on the tongue or forehead. For these thermometers follow the manufacturers instructions. If you only have an 'old fashioned' mercury thermometer however, the following advice may help:

- Take care when handling the thermometer. The mercury centre is poisonous.
- Ensure that it has been properly cleaned.
- Hold the thermometer at the opposite end to the silver mercury bulb.
- Shake the thermometer until the mercury falls well below the 35°C mark.
- Place under the tongue of an adult *(who is fully conscious),* or the armpit of a child.
- Keep in place for 3 minutes.
- Read the temperature at the level to which the mercury has risen.

the digestive system

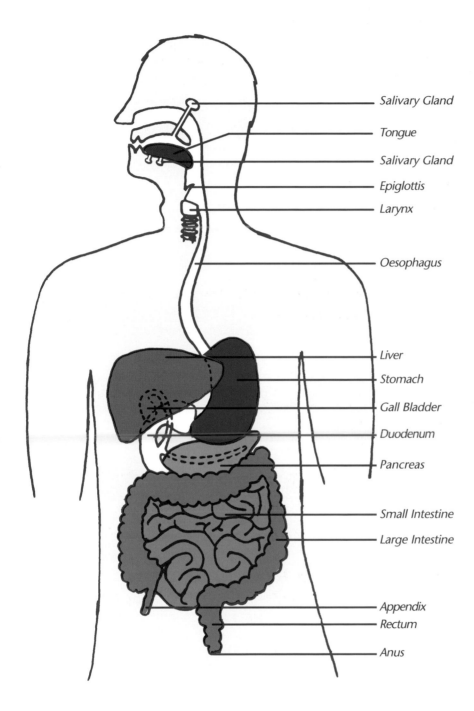

Salivary Gland

Tongue

Salivary Gland

Epiglottis

Larynx

Oesophagus

Liver

Stomach

Gall Bladder

Duodenum

Pancreas

Small Intestine

Large Intestine

Appendix

Rectum

Anus

Food enters the body through the mouth, where it is mechanically broken down by chewing, and the salivary glands secrete saliva, which helps break down starches (amongst other substances).

As we swallow, the epiglottis folds down to prevent food entering the airway, and the 'bolus' of food enters the oesophagus.

The bolus of food is pushed through the oesophagus (and the rest of the digestive system) by waves of muscle contractions.

Food enters the stomach, where acidic gastric juices are secreted to help break down the bolus of food to a soup like consistency.

The food then enters the duodenum, which is a duct into which enzymes from the pancreas, gall bladder and liver are secreted. These enzymes enable food to be broken down further, as it continues into the small intestine.

Although it is called the 'small' intestine, this duct is around 5 metres in length, and coils around in the centre of the abdominal cavity.
The small intestine completes the digestion process by absorbing nutrients from the food into the blood stream for use by the body.

Undigested food now passes into the large intestine (colon), where water is absorbed into the body, before being excreted from the anus.

Up to 1 minute

30 seconds

2 to 4 hours

2 to 6 hours

10 hours to several days

diabetes

Diabetes is the name for a condition suffered by a person who does not produce enough of a hormone called insulin.

Insulin breaks down the sugar that we digest, so that it can be used by the cells of the body or stored for later use. In summary, insulin reduces the amount of sugar in the blood.

If diabetes goes untreated, the level of sugar in the blood will climb dangerously high over 1 to 2 days *(depending on the severity of the condition)*.

There are 3 different types of diabetes, which are categorised by their method of treatment:

Diet Controlled This patient still produces some insulin naturally, so can control the condition by reducing the amount of sugar that they eat.

Tablet Controlled This patient still produces a small amount of insulin naturally, but needs to take tablets to help reduce the level of sugar in the blood, as well as diet control.

Insulin Dependent This patient produces little or no insulin, and has to inject themselves with insulin 2 or more times a day in order to keep sugar levels under control.

high blood sugar - (hyper*glycaemia*)

Hyperglycaemia is the condition that occurs if diabetes has not been treated effectively with the methods mentioned above.

The sugar levels in the blood become higher and acids build up. The signs and symptoms in the table *(opposite)* are as a direct result of the body trying to excrete this acid build up.

low blood sugar - (hypo*glycaemia*)

Low blood sugar occurs mainly with diabetic patients who are insulin dependent, because the level of insulin in the body is now a 'fixed' amount because it is injected.

Because the patient has injected this 'fixed' amount of insulin, they have to balance it with the amount of food that they eat.

The blood sugar levels will fall low if:

- The patient does not eat enough food.

- The patient over exercises *(burning off sugar)*.

- The patient injects too much insulin.

why is low blood sugar dangerous?

Unlike other cells in the body, the brain can only use glucose *(sugar)* as its source of energy. If the sugar in the blood becomes low therefore, the brain cells are literally starved.

The signs and symptoms of low blood sugar in the table *(opposite)* are as a result of the hungry brain cells becoming disordered, and the release of adrenaline that the disorder in the brain causes. *(see also 'the body's response to hypoxia'- page 14).*

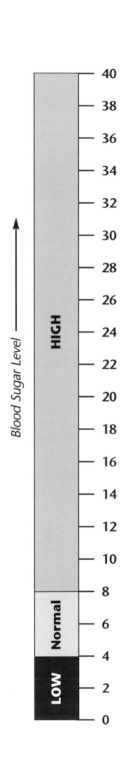

Blood Sugar Level

HIGH — 40, 38, 36, 34, 32, 30, 28, 26, 24, 22, 20, 18, 16, 14, 12, 10, 8

Normal — 8, 6, 4

LOW — 4, 2, 0

possible signs and symptoms

	High Blood Sugar (hyperglycaemia)	Low Blood Sugar (hypoglycaemia)
Onset	Slow – 12 to 48 hours	Fast – 2 minutes to 1 hour
Levels of Response	Deteriorate slowly during the onset: • Drowsy, lethargic behaviour • Unconsciousness if the condition is left untreated	Deteriorate rapidly: • Weakness, dizziness • Confusion, memory loss • Lack of coordination • Slurred speech • Bizarre, uncharacteristic, uncooperative, possibly violent behaviour • Unconsciousness within 1 hour
Skin	Dry and warm	Pale, cold and sweaty
Breathing	Deep sighing breaths	Normal, or shallow and rapid
Pulse	Rapid	Rapid
Other Symptoms	Excessive urination Excessive thirst Hunger Fruity odour on the breath	Beware – the signs and symptoms can be confused for drunkenness

treatment of high blood sugar

• Arrange for the patient to see a doctor as soon as possible.

• If the patient becomes unconscious, maintain **Airway** and **Breathing**, and **dial 999 for an ambulance** *(see pages 6 to 8)*.

treatment of low blood sugar

for a conscious casualty:

• Sit the casualty down.

• Give the casualty a sugary drink *(isotonic sports drinks are best)*, sugar lumps, glucose tablets, chocolate, or other sweet foods.

• If the casualty responds to treatment quickly, give them more food or drink.

• Stay with the casualty and let them rest until the level of response is 'fully alert' *(see page 9)*.

• Tell the patient to see their doctor – even though they have fully recovered.

• If the patient does not respond to treatment within 10 minutes, or they are unmanageable, **dial 999 for an ambulance.**

• Consider if there is another cause for the patient's symptoms.

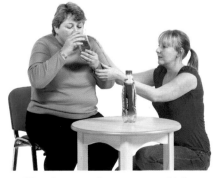

Give the casualty a sugary drink – isotonic sports drinks are best.

for an unconscious casualty:

• Open the **Airway** and check for **Breathing**. Resuscitate as necessary *(pages 6 to 8)*.

• Place the casualty in the recovery position if they are breathing effectively.

• **Dial 999 for an ambulance.**

other serious conditions

poisons

A poison can be described as any substance *(solid, liquid or gas)* that causes damage when it enters the body in a sufficient quantity.

Poisons can enter the body in 4 ways, they can be:

Ingested   Swallowed, either accidentally or on purpose.

Inhaled   Breathed in, accessing the blood stream very quickly as it passes through the alveoli.

Absorbed   Through the skin *(see chemical burns, page 33)*.

Injected   Through the skin, directly into tissues or a blood vessel.

A poison can either be:

Corrosive   Such as: acids, bleach, ammonia, petrol, turpentine, dishwasher powder, etc.

Non-Corrosive Such as: tablets, drugs, alcohol, plants, perfume etc.

possible signs and symptoms   ?

The signs and symptoms of poisoning are wide, varied and dependent on the substance. Look for clues such as:

- Containers or bottles.
- Tablets or drugs.
- Syringe or drug taking equipment.
- Smell on the breath.

other signs that can accompany poisoning may be:

- Vomiting or retching.
- Abdominal pains.
- Burns *(or burning sensation)* around the entry area.
- Breathing problems.
- Confusion or hallucination.
- Headache.
- Unconsciousness, sometimes fitting.
- Cyanosis.

treatment   ✚

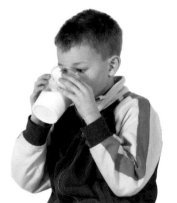

Get the casualty to rinse out their mouth, then give frequent sips of milk or water.

for a corrosive substance:

- Don't endanger yourself – make sure it's safe to help.
- Dilute the substance or wash it away if possible:
  - Substances on the skin – see chemical burns *(page 33)*.
  - Ingested Substances – get the casualty to rinse out their mouth, then give frequent sips of milk or water.
- **Dial 999 for an ambulance.** Give information about the poison if possible. Take advice from the ambulance operator.
- If the casualty becomes unconscious – open the **Airway** and check for **Breathing**. Resuscitate as necessary using a protective face-shield *(pages 6 to 8)*. If the casualty is breathing effectively, place them in the recovery position, then **dial 999 for an ambulance.**

for a non-corrosive substance:

- **Dial 999 for an ambulance.** Give information about the poison if possible. Take advice from the ambulance operator.
- If the casualty becomes unconscious –- open the **Airway** and check for **Breathing**. Resuscitate as necessary using a protective face-shield *(pages 6 to 8)*. If the casualty is breathing effectively, place them in the recovery position, then **dial 999 for an ambulance.**

NEVER make the patient vomit. This may put the airway in danger.

It helps the Paramedics if you:

- *Pass on containers, or other information about the substance.*
- *Find out how much has been taken.*
- *Find out when it was taken.*
- *Keep samples of any vomit for hospital analysis.*

epilepsy

A person diagnosed with epilepsy has a tendency to have recurrent seizures *(fits)* that arise from a disturbance in the brain. This chapter does not only deal with patients who are diagnosed with epilepsy however, because one person in 20 will have a seizure at some point in their lives.

There are many causes of fitting *(including epilepsy)*, such as hypoxia, stroke, head injury or even the body's temperature becoming too high.

Babies and young children commonly suffer fits from becoming too hot due to illness and fever. This is covered in the topic 'febrile convulsions', overleaf.

minor seizures

Minor epilepsy is also known as 'absence seizures' or 'petit mal' fits. The patient may appear to suddenly start day dreaming *(even mid sentence)*. This may last just a few seconds before recovery, and the patient might not even realise what has happened. Sometimes a minor fit may be accompanied by strange movements, such as twitching the face, jerking of an individual limb, or lip smacking. The patient may make a noise, such as letting out a cry.

treatment of minor seizures

- Remove any sources of danger, such as a knife or hot drink in their hands.
- Help the patient to sit down in a quiet place and reassure them.
- Stay with the patient until they are fully alert *(page 9)*.
- If the patient is unaware of their condition, advise them to see a doctor.

major seizures

This type of seizure results from a major disturbance in the brain, which causes aggressive fitting, usually of the whole body.

Witnessing a major fit can be frightening for the first aider, but calm, prompt action is essential for the patient.

possible signs and symptoms

A major fit usually goes through a pattern:

Aura If the patient has had fits before, they may recognise that they are about to have one. The warning sign may be anything from a strange taste in the mouth, a smell, or a peculiar feeling. The aura may give the patient chance to seek help, or simply lie down before they fall.

'Tonic' Phase Every muscle in the body suddenly becomes rigid. The patient may let out a cry and will fall to the floor. The back may arch and the lips may go blue *(cyanosis)*. This phase typically lasts less than 20 seconds.

'Clonic' Phase The limbs of the body make sudden, violent jerking movements, the eyes may roll, the teeth may clench, saliva may drool from the mouth *(sometimes blood-stained as a result of biting the tongue)* and breathing could be loud like 'snoring'. The patient may lose control of the bladder or bowel.

This phase can last from 30 seconds to hours, although most fits stop within a couple of minutes. Any fit *(or series of fits)* lasting more than 15 minutes is a dire medical emergency.

Recovery Phase The body relaxes, though the patient is still unresponsive. Levels of response *(page 9)* will improve within a few minutes, but the patient may not be 'fully alert' for 20 minutes or so. They may be unaware of their actions and might want to sleep to recuperate.

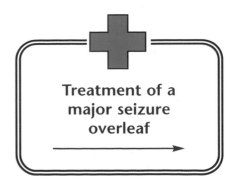

Treatment of a major seizure overleaf

treatment of major seizures *(fitting)*

during the seizure:

- Help the patient to the floor to avoid injury if possible.

- Gently cushion the patient's head to help avoid injury. This can be done simply with your hands or a folded coat.

- Loosen any tight clothing around the neck to help the patient breathe.

- Move any objects from around the patient that may harm them and ask bystanders to move away.

- If you are concerned about the **Airway**, roll the casualty onto their side.

- Take note of the exact time the fitting started and its duration.

- Look for identification if you don't know the patient.

dial 999 for an ambulance if:

- The fitting lasts more than 3 minutes.

- The patient's levels of response *(page 9)* don't improve after the fit within 10 minutes.

- The patient has a second fit.

- The patient is not diagnosed as epileptic or this is their first fit.

- You are unsure.

as soon as the fitting stops:

- Check **Airway** and **Breathing**. Resuscitate if necessary *(pages 6 to 8)*.

- Place the patient in the recovery position *(page 12)*.

- Keep the patient warm *(unless temperature caused the fit)* and reassure them.

- Monitor **Airway** and **Breathing**.

- Move bystanders away before the casualty awakes and protect modesty.

- Check the levels of response regularly *(page 9)*. **Dial 999** if they don't improve within 10 minutes *(or for any of the reasons mentioned above)*.

febrile convulsions

In young children and babies the area of the brain that regulates temperature *(the hypothalamus)* is not yet fully developed. This can lead to the core temperature of the body reaching dangerously high levels *(page 41)* and commonly a child in this situation may fit.

A febrile convulsion can be very frightening for the parents of the child. During the 'tonic' phase of the fit *(page 49)* the child may stop breathing, because the diaphragm goes rigid, and the lips and face may go blue *(cyanosis)*. It goes without saying therefore, that calm reassurance will be necessary.

The child may have been unwell over the past day or so and will be hot to touch.

treatment of febrile convulsions

- Remove clothing and bedclothes. Provide fresh, cool air to cool the child down. Take care not to cool the child too much.

- Place the child on their side if possible to protect the **Airway**.

- Remove nearby objects and use padding to protect the child from injury whilst fitting. Pay particular attention to protecting the head.

- **Dial 999 for an ambulance.**

- Sponge the child with tepid water to help the cooling process.

- Constantly monitor **Airway** and **Breathing** until the ambulance arrives.

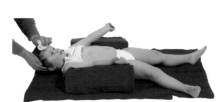

Gently protect the head.

NEVER place anything in the casualty's mouth *(especially your fingers!)*.

NEVER try to hold the patient down or restrain them.

NEVER move the casualty *(unless they are in danger)*.

Protect the child from injury and sponge with tepid water to help the cooling process.

moving and handling

Moving and handling a human being is much more difficult than it appears, especially if that person is unconscious *(and therefore very floppy)*.

For this reason, you should never attempt to move a casualty unless it is absolutely necessary. You may harm the patient and injure yourself.

If you have no other option than to move a patient however, following the rules and methods in this chapter should reduce the risk of injury.

moving and handling rules

before the move, THINK:

- Can the casualty move themselves? Is there another option to lifting them? Will it make their condition worse if they walk?

- How heavy is the patient? Do you need more help?

- Is the route clear and safe? *(you can't move furniture at the same time as carrying someone!)*

- Is there any equipment that you can utilise to help you?
  Are you *(or is someone else)* trained to use it?

during the move, ensure that you and others:

- Stand as close to the patient as possible *(don't stretch out)*.

- Bend with your knees, not your back.

- Keep your back upright, but not rigid.

- Use your most powerful muscles *(your legs, not your back!)*.

- Take your time. Rushing will injure you.

- Talk to your helpers – so that you move together as a team. One person should take charge.

Here are some principles that should be followed whenever you attempt to move or lift an object:

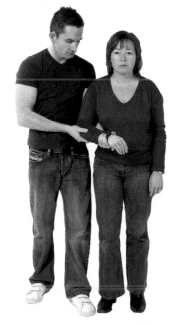

Helping a casualty to walk:

- *Place your arm under theirs, and take a firm hold of their wrist.*

- *Hold their elbow with your opposite arm.*

- *If the casualty begins to pass out, do not try to hold them up as this may injure you – carefully lower them to the floor instead (see overleaf).*

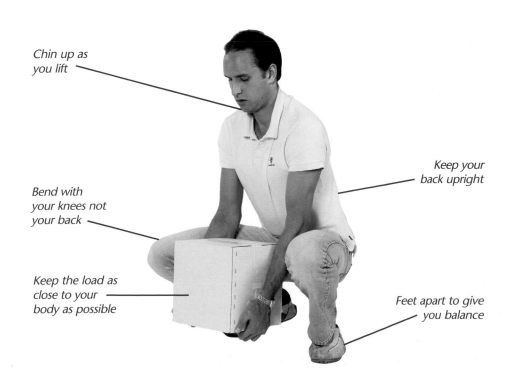

Chin up as you lift

Keep your back upright

Bend with your knees not your back

Keep the load as close to your body as possible

Feet apart to give you balance

More methods of moving a casualty overleaf →

health and safety

methods of moving

IMPORTANT: *See notes on moving and handling – previous page.*

lowering from chair to floor:

This manoeuvre can be made easier by using a moving aid called a 'slide sheet'. This is a low friction sheet which can be placed under the patient's buttocks to make sliding them easier.

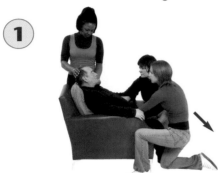

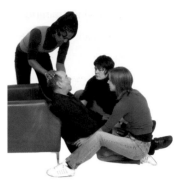

Helper 1:

- Support the patient's head throughout the manoeuvre.

Helpers 2 and 3:

- Place your outer foot on the floor. Kneel with your inner leg.
- With your inner arm, hold the back of the patient's leg, just above the knee.
- With your outer arm, grasp the patient's waist line *(or the slide sheet)*.

Helpers 2 and 3:

- Keeping your foot and knee in the same position on the floor, lean backwards, sliding the patient to the floor.
- Remove the chair to lower the patient's head to the floor.
- If you can't move the chair, perform the manoeuvre again to slide the patient further onto the floor.

controlling a fall:

If a patient begins to pass out, do not try to hold them up as this may injure you.

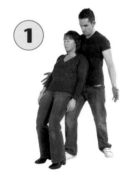

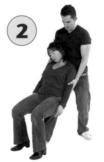

- Release your hold slightly and move behind the patient.
- Place your feet shoulder width apart to give you balance.

- Allow the patient to slide down your body as you stay in an upright posture.

blanket lift:

This manoeuvre is best if you use a 'carry sheet', which is designed for lifting a patient. If you don't have enough helpers, another option is to drag the patient on the sheet, instead of lifting them.

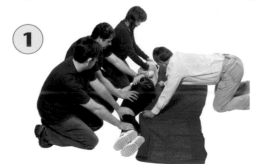

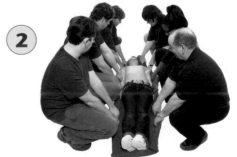

- Turn the patient onto one side.
- Roll one edge of a blanket and place it behind them.

- Turn the patient over the rolled edge, onto their back.
- Roll the open edge of the blanket up.
- Use the rolls at either side of the patient to lift with.

health and safety (first aid) regulations 1981

employer's responsibilities

Under Health and Safety law, an employer has a responsibility to ensure that first aid provision in the workplace is sufficient. This includes:

- Carrying out an assessment to decide how many First Aiders are needed and where they should be located, following guidance from the Health and Safety Executive.
- Providing training and re-qualifying training for those First Aiders.
- Providing sufficient first aid kits and equipment for the workplace.
- Ensuring that all staff are aware of how and where to get first aid treatment.

This chapter gives some guidance on these responsibilities, although first aid training organisations are always willing to give advice.

first aid kits

First Aid kits should be easily accessible and clearly identified by a white cross on a green background. The container should protect the contents from dust and damp.

A first aid kit should be available at every work site. Larger sites may need more than one first aid kit. The following list of contents is given as guidance:

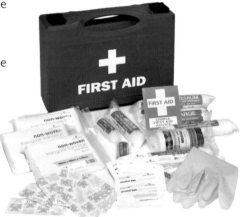

- A leaflet giving general guidance on first aid.
- 20 individually wrapped sterile adhesive dressings of assorted size *(plasters)*. Blue detectable plasters should be provided for food handlers.
- 2 sterile eye pads.
- 4 triangular bandages, individually wrapped and preferably sterile.
- 6 safety pins.
- 6 medium wound dressings *(approx. 12cm x 12cm)*, individually wrapped and sterile.
- 2 large wound dressings *(approx. 18cm x 18cm)*, as above.
- 1 pair of disposable gloves.

The list is not mandatory, so equivalent items may be used. Other items such as scissors, adhesive tape or disposable aprons should be provided if necessary. They may be stored in the first aid kit if they will fit, or kept close by for use.

Other items that may need to be considered are such things as blankets to protect casualties from the elements, or protective equipment such as breathing apparatus if a First Aider had to enter a dangerous atmosphere.

eye wash

If mains tap water is not readily available for eye irrigation, at least 1 litre of sterile water or 'saline' should be provided in sealed disposable container*(s)*.

travelling first aid kits

First Aid kits for travelling workers should typically include:

- A leaflet giving general guidance on first aid.
- 6 individually wrapped sterile adhesive dressings of assorted size *(plasters)*.
- 1 large wound dressing *(approx. 18cm x 18cm)*.
- 2 triangular bandages.
- 2 safety pins.
- Individually wrapped moist cleansing wipes.
- 1 pair of disposable gloves.

health and safety

first aiders

The selection of a First Aider depends upon a number of factors. The person best suited to be a First Aider will volunteer, and will have:

- good reliability, disposition and communication skills.

- an aptitude and ability to absorb new skills and knowledge.

- an ability to cope with stressful and physically demanding emergency procedures.

- normal duties in the workplace that can be left, to respond immediately and rapidly to an emergency.

number of first aiders required

The table below, compiled using information from the Health and Safety Executive, gives an indication of the number of First Aiders required in the work place:

Risk Category	Number of Employees	Suggested Number of First Aiders
Lower Risk e.g. shops, offices, libraries.	Fewer than 50	At least 1 Appointed Person
	50 to 100	At least 1 First Aider
	More than 100	1 additional First Aider for every 100 employed
Medium Risk e.g. light engineering, assembly work, food processing, warehousing.	Fewer than 20	At least 1 Appointed Person
	20 to 100	At least 1 First Aider for every 50 employed (or part thereof)
	More than 100	1 additional First Aider for every 100 employed
Higher Risk e.g. construction work, slaughter houses, chemical manufacture, work with dangerous machinery or sharp instruments.	Fewer than 5	At least 1 Appointed Person
	5 to 50	At least 1 First Aider
	More than 50	1 additional First Aider for every 50 employed

The numbers given in the table are minimum requirements. You should then add First Aiders to take account of the following:

- **Foreseeable absences** – cover should remain adequate even when First Aiders are absent on such occasions as annual leave.

- **Shift Work** – every shift should be adequately covered.

- **Large Sites** – First Aiders should be in close proximity to all areas.

- **Isolated Work Locations** – Cover should be provided if necessary.

Finally, Health and Safety at Work Regulations do not take account of non-employees *(such as your customers)*.

The Health and Safety Executive do, however **Strongly Recommend** that you take non-employees into account when assessing the need for first aid requirements. You should certainly consider the liability implications if you do not!

appointed persons

Where an employer's assessment of first aid requirements identifies that a First Aider is not necessary, the minimum requirement on the employer is to appoint a person to take charge of first aid arrangements, including looking after equipment and facilities and taking charge in an emergency situation. An appointed person should be available to undertake these duties at all times when people are at work.

Training courses for Appointed Persons are approximately 4 or 8 hours in duration, and cover:

- What to do in an emergency.
- Cardio Pulmonary Resuscitation.
- First Aid for the unconscious casualty.
- First Aid for wounds and bleeding.
- Dealing with common medical conditions.

first aider

A First Aider is a person who has been trained by, and holds a current certificate of an organisation whose training and qualifications are approved by the Health and Safety Executive.

First Aiders are trained to deal with the majority of emergency situations that can occur in the workplace, but may require extra training if special conditions exist at work, *(e.g. use of breathing equipment if they might have to enter a dangerous atmosphere to administer first aid).*

First Aid certificates issued by such organisations are valid for 3 years and the First Aider must re-qualify before the certificate expires.

Training courses for a First Aid at Work qualification are 4 days in duration.

Re-qualification courses are 2 days in duration, but must be taken before the first aid certificate expires or the candidate has to attend a full 4 day course.

reporting of incidents at work

Any accident at work, no matter how small, must be recorded in an accident book *(see overleaf)*. The incident may also need to be reported directly to the Health and Safety Executive under RIDDOR regulations:

RIDDOR 1995 regulations

Reporting of **I**njuries, **D**iseases and **D**angerous **O**ccurrences **R**egulations 1995.

These regulations state that it is the responsibility of the *Employer* to report the following occurrences directly to the Health and Safety Executive:

- Deaths.
- Major injuries.
- Accidents resulting in 3 or more days off work.
- Diseases.
- Dangerous occurrences.

For more information you can visit the RIDDOR web site at: www.riddor.gov.uk

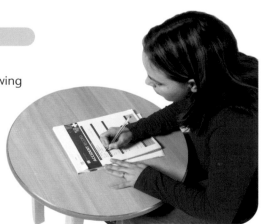

accident book

Any accident at work, no matter how small, must be recorded in an accident book. The accident book may be filled in by any person on behalf of the casualty *(or indeed by the casualty themselves)*.

The information recorded can help the employer identify accident trends and possible areas of improvement in the control of health and safety risks. It can be used for future first aid needs assessments and may be helpful for insurance investigative purposes.

Filling in the accident book is often done by the First Aider, so the following notes are given for your advice:

- An accident book is a legal document.
- Anything that has been written down at the time of an incident is usually considered to be 'stronger evidence' in court than something recalled from memory.
- Complete the report all at the same time, using the same pen *(not pencil)*.
- To comply with the Data Protection Act, personal details entered in accident books must be kept confidential, so the book should be designed so that individual record sheets can be removed and stored securely.
- A member of staff should be nominated to be responsible for the safekeeping of completed accident records *(e.g. in a lockable cabinet)*. Hand the completed accident record to that person.
- The person who had the accident may wish to take a photocopy of the report. If this is the case, they can do this before it is handed in. They should keep a record of the accident report number.

you should include in the report:

- The name, address and occupation of the person who had the accident.
- The name, address, occupation and signature of the person who is completing the report.
- The date, time and location of the accident.
- A description of how the accident happened, giving the cause if you can.
- Details of the injury suffered.

A typical accident record form.

first aid patient report form

It is useful for a first aider to complete a patient report form for every patient treated. Please note that this does not replace the accident book, which would still have to be completed for an accident at work.

A copy of a patient report form is opposite. You can make copies of this for your own use.

The patient report form is designed so the first aider can keep a record of the exact treatment provided. It is particularly useful if a patient refuses treatment against the advice of the first aider.

- If a patient refuses treatment, make sure they are capable of making that decision *(e.g. a fully conscious adult)*. Seek medical advice if they are not.
- Follow the advice given for completing the accident book *(above)* when completing the form.
- A copy of the form can be given to ambulance or hospital staff, as it will contain valuable information about the incident and treatment of the patient. Ask the nurse to take a copy, so you can keep the original.
- To comply with the Data Protection Act, personal details on the report form must be kept confidential, so the report should be stored securely *(e.g. in a lockable cabinet)*.

AVPU score

A simple way to record the conscious level of a patient is to use the 'AVPU' scale. A detailed explanation of the scale is given on page 9.

The scale is listed on the patient report form so you don't have to remember it. There is a score provided next to each level of consciousness. Write the score in the observations chart each time you measure it.

first aid patient report form

Date _____ Time _____ First Aider _____

Patient Name _____ Sex _____ Date of Birth _____ Age _____

Patient's Address _____

Location of Incident _____

Patient Observations: *(record at least every 10 minutes)*

Time			Breathing Rate		Pulse Rate		AVPU SCORE

AVPU SCORE:		SCORE:
Alert	Fully Alert (usually knows the month).	6
Voice	Confused.	5
	Inappropriate Words.	4
	Utters Sounds.	3
Pain	Localises Pain.	2
	Responds to (but does not localise) Pain	1
Unresponsive	Unresponsive to speech and pain stimuli.	0

A.M.P.L.E.

Allergies	
Medication	
Past Medical History	
Last Eaten	
Events Leading to Incident	
Treatment / Comments	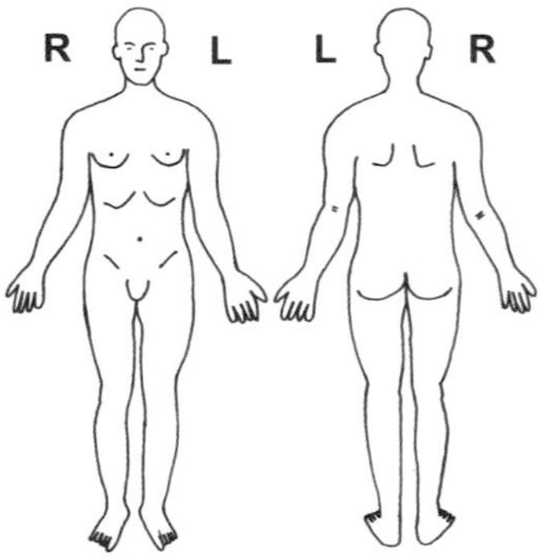

Patient's Signature: _____   Date: _____

First Aider's Signature: _____   Date: _____

Abdomen	The area between the lowest ribs and the pelvis.
Acute	Sudden onset.
Adrenaline	Hormone secreted by the body in times of shock (see page 14).
...aem...	Referring to the blood.
Airway	The passage from the mouth and nose to the lungs.
Alveoli	Minute air sacks in the lungs, through which the exchange of gases takes place.
Asphyxia	Deficiency of oxygen caused by an interruption in the passage of air to the lungs.
Atrium	Top, 'collecting' chamber of the heart (of which there are two).
Baby	Person under 1 year old.
Breathing	Inspiration and expiration of air into and out of the lungs.
Bronchioles	Small air passages in the lungs, leading to the alveoli.
Cardiac / cardiogenic	Concerned with the heart.
Cell	Smallest structural living unit of an organism.
Cerebro-spinal fluid (CSF)	Fluid that surrounds the brain and spinal cord, to cushion it and provide nutrients etc.
Cerebrum	The largest part of the brain.
Cervical	Concerned with the neck.
Child	Person between 1 year old and puberty.
Chronic	Long term.
Circulation	The movement of blood around the body.
Compression	Bleeding or swelling in the cranial cavity, exerting pressure on the brain.
Concussion	Shaking of the brain, causing temporary loss of consciousness or function.
Consciousness	Alertness, 'normal' activity of the brain.
Constrict	To close down, become narrower.
Convulsion	Fit or Seizure.
CPR	Cardio Pulmonary Resuscitation. Manually squeezing the heart and breathing for a patient.
Cranium	The cavity in the skull in which the brain lies.
Cyanosis	Blue grey tinges to the skin, especially the lips, due to lack of oxygen.
Defibrillation	The delivery of a large electric shock to the chest in an attempt to re-start the heart.
Dilate	Become wider, open up.
Enzyme	Substance that enables a biological reaction to happen.
Epistaxis	Nose bleed.
Febrile	Relating to fever or high body temperature.
Haemothorax	Bleeding into the pleural cavity of the lungs.
Hepatic	Relating to the liver.
Hyper...	High.

Hypo...	Low.
Hypothalamus	Area of the brain that controls body temperature.
Hypovolaemic	Low volume of blood, a type of shock.
Hypoxia	Low levels of oxygen in the blood.
Inferior	Below.
Insulin	Hormone secreted by the pancreas that enables the usage and storage of sugar.
Jaw Thrust	Manoeuvre to open the airway without moving the head, by thrusting the jaw forwards.
Mesenteric	Relating to an area of the intestines.
Nausea	Feeling sick.
Neurogenic	Concerned with the brain and nervous system.
Perfusion	Supply of oxygen and nutrients, and the removal of waste gases and products.
Pleura	A two layered membrane surrounding the lungs, between which is a 'serous' fluid.
Pneumothorax	Air entry into the pleural cavity of the lung.
Pulmonary	Concerned with the lungs.
Regurgitation	Vomiting, being sick.
Rescue Breath	Blowing air into a patient's lungs, sufficient to make the chest rise.
Respiration	Breathing.
Resusci-aid	Protective mask with a one-way valve for performing mouth-to-mouth rescue breaths.
Seizure	Fit or Convulsion.
Shock	Inadequate supply of oxygen to the tissues as a result of a fall in blood pressure or volume.
Spinal cord	Group of nerves which emanate from the brain and pass down the spinal column.
Spine	The column of vertebrae which form the back.
Stroke	Bleed or blockage of a blood vessel within the brain (see page 13).
Superior	Above.
Symptoms	The feelings of a patient e.g. "I feel sick."
Syncope	Faint.
Tension pneumothorax	Air entry into the pleural cavity of the lung that has become pressurised, impairing the function of the good lung and the heart.
Thoracic	The area within the rib cage containing the lungs.
Tourniquet	A tight band placed around a limb which was used to stop blood flow. No longer used in first aid.
Ventricle	Lower, larger 'pumping' chamber of the heart (of which there are two).
Ventricular Fibrillation	Quivering, vibrating movement of the ventricles of the heart, producing no effective pumping action.

notes

The following questions are provided so you can test your knowledge of first aid. **Discuss with your first aid instructor which questions are best to revise**. Write your answers on a separate sheet of paper.

Answer the questions as best as you can from memory, then have a look in the book to mark yourself *(or improve your answers)*. *The page numbers in italics indicate where to look for the correct answer.*

1.   What is the order of priorities when dealing with a patient?
     Page 4

2.   What ratio of chest compressions to rescue breaths would you do when performing CPR?
     Page 7

3.   What modifications can you make to the adult sequence of CPR to make it even more suitable for a child?
     Page 8

4.   What are the 2 main dangers facing someone who is unconscious and on their back?
     Page 11

5.   How would you treat a patient who is unconscious because of head injury?
     Page 13

6.   What are the signs and symptoms of hypoxia?
     Page 14

7.   Try to remember as many of the causes of hypoxia as you can.
     Page 14

8.   Someone starts to choke on some food. What should you do?
     Pages 16 or 17

9.   Someone is suffering from anaphylaxis shock and they are struggling to breathe. How will they look?
     Page 18

10. How would you treat a patient having an asthma attack?
     Page 19

11. What are the average pulse rates of: a) an adult.   b) a child.   c) a baby.
     Page 23

12. What are the signs and symptoms of a heart attack?
     Page 24

13. How would you treat a patient suffering from heart attack?
     Page 25

14. Someone has cut their arm on some sharp metal. The metal isn't stuck in the wound but it is bleeding badly. What should you do?
     Page 30

15. Someone in the kitchen has slipped with a sharp knife and amputated their finger. Describe your actions.
     Pages 30 and 31

16. Someone has scalded the whole of their hand on some hot water. What should you do? What percentage of burn is that?
     Pages 33 and 34

17. Can you remember some signs and symptoms of a fracture?
     Page 37

18. A patient has fractured their wrist. How would you treat the patient?
     Page 37

19. A patient has fallen from a horse and they are unconscious. You check breathing and they are breathing normally. What should you do now?
     Page 39

20. Someone has been working outside in very cold rainy weather all day. You suspect they are hypothermic. How should you treat them?
     Page 42

21. A diabetic patient is suddenly acting strangely and not making sense. What is probably wrong? What should you do?
     Pages 46 and 47

22. How would you treat a patient having an epileptic fit? What should you do after they have stopped fitting?
     Page 50